Trauma Center Performance Improvement

Jeffrey S. Young

Trauma Center Performance Improvement

Principles and Practice, With Illustrative
Case Studies

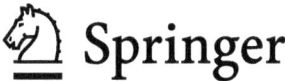 Springer

Jeffrey S. Young
Acute Care Surgery
University of Virginia
Charlottesville, VA
USA

ISBN 978-3-030-71047-7   ISBN 978-3-030-71048-4   (eBook)
https://doi.org/10.1007/978-3-030-71048-4

This Springer imprint is published by the registered company Springer Nature Switzerland AG
The registered company address is: Gewerbestrasse 11, 6330 Cham, Switzerland

This work is dedicated to all the pre-hospital, emergency department, operating room, intensive care unit, acute care, and rehabilitation personnel who care for the injured patient.

Preface

Managing a trauma center is the most difficult role a surgeon can play. It involves complex clinical care, long nights and days, administrative work, self-examination and critical review of patient care, and significant regulatory requirements. Performance improvement is the key element of trauma center effectiveness. No trauma center provides flawless care, thus all centers have opportunities to improve. Deficits in the PI process are the most cited deficiency in American College of Surgeons site visits, and the Society of Trauma Nurses has provided an outstanding framework for a PI program in their Trauma Outcomes and Improvement Course. This book is meant to expand on the information they provide to help programs better understand the PI process. This book is not approved by the STN or the American College of Surgeons, but I have spent 16 years site visiting trauma centers, as well as running my own trauma center for 26 years. Thus, I feel I have some useful information to impart.

In this book, I have attempted to provide key information on all aspects of trauma PI program management. In some ways, PI is an art more than a science, so the more interaction program leaders have with strong PI programs, the more they can learn about how to improve their processes.

Any of the chapters or sections of this work can be read independently; however, a physician or TPM leading a trauma center should read as much of the entire book as possible since it will help them understand the entirety of the PI process.

Charlottesville, VA, USA   Jeffrey S. Young

Acknowledgments

I would like to thank Kathy Butler, Michelle Pomphrey, Sera Downing, Val Quick, Shannon Critzer, Avis Brent, Amy Bunts, and Forrest Calland for their untiring assistance with running a trauma center. But most importantly I would like to thank my wife Denise and my children Andy, Steven, Brian, Erin, Leigh, Yogi, Butter, and Decimus for their support and love.

Abbreviations

ABC	Airway, breathing and circulation
ACS	American College of Surgeons
COT	Committee on Trauma
CT	Computed tomography
EAST	Eastern Association for the Surgery of Trauma
ED	Emergency department
EMT	Emergency medical technician
GCS	Glasgow coma score
GSW	Gunshot wound
ICU	Intensive care unit
IEP	Internal education program
LMA	Laryngeal mask airway
M&M	Morbidity and mortality conference
MDPI	Multidisciplinary Performance Improvement Committee
MRI	Magnetic resonance imaging
MTP	Massive transfusion protocol
OFI	Opportunity for improvement
PI	Performance improvement
POS	Probability of survival
PRQ	Pre-review questionnaire
SICU	Surgical Intensive Care Unit
STN	Society of trauma nurses
TMD	Trauma Medical Director
TOPIC	Trauma outcomes and performant improvement course
TPM	Trauma Program Manager
TQIP	Trauma quality improvement project

Contents

About the Author

Jeffrey S. Young, MD, MBA was born in Brooklyn, New York, and attended the University of Virginia, Medical College of Virginia, and trained in trauma and general surgery at Wake Forest University under the mentorship of Dr. J. Wayne Meredith. He assumed the role of trauma director of the University of Virginia (UVA) trauma center in July 1994 and has held that role since.

Dr. Young is a former member of the National Committee on Trauma, and is currently a Chief of Region III for the American College of Surgeons (ACS) Committee on Trauma (COT). He is a former associate chief of staff, chief quality officer, chief patient safety officer, and medical director of the Surgical Subspecialties Service Line at UVA. He has published over 90 peer-reviewed articles on trauma care and is a tenured professor of surgery and division chief of acute care surgery. Dr. Young has been a member of the ACS COT Verification Review Committee since 1998 and has performed over 180 trauma center site visits for the ACS, as well as for the states of Maryland and Oregon.

His wife Denise is an associate professor of obstetrics and gynecology. He has five children and three dogs. Andy is a general surgery resident at UVA, Steven is a fourth-year medical student at UVA, Brian is a student at James Madison University (JMU) and a paramedic, his daughter Erin is a sophomore at UVA, and his daughter Leigh is a high school student and top-flight lacrosse player who will be playing Division I Lacrosse at the University of Pittsburgh. He lives in Troy, Virginia.

Chapter 1
What Is PI? (and What It Is Not)

Why PI?

Medicine has had a long and not always laudable history of attempting to improve itself. Since healthcare is a skill set possessed by only a small number of practitioners, outside "interference" in clinical practice was not well received. The long years of training and long hours spent caring for patients ingrained a sense of omniscience to many practitioners, even though it was easy for them to see another doctor in the same specialty practicing entirely differently, and both doctors thinking their way was the best. Thus, improvement in care may be stimulated from outside forces but can only occur from the inside out.

This strong outside influence came in the form of a report by the Institute for Healthcare Improvement in 2000 [1]. This report provided evidence that American healthcare was not safe in many hospitals, that serious errors were occurring, and that there were little to no action-oriented improvement processes in many facilities. It provided a framework for performance improvement.

Trauma centers have been leaders in performance improvement for decades. This originated from the efforts in Orange County, California, spearheaded by trauma surgeons in that region. These nascent activities included chart review discussion of adverse events and deaths and group discussions, bringing together surgeons from many hospitals to discuss their cases. From this grew efforts to codify performance improvement principles including monitoring, issue identification, analysis, the formation of countermeasures, implementation of corrective action plans, and auditing to ensure that the problem was solved. There is a great deal of interest in literature written about performance improvement and patient safety in the surgical domain. I invite the readers to look at these textbooks since they provide a great deal of information. The purpose of this text is to provide a practical guide for performance improvement and to provide examples of the performance improvement process.

© The Author(s), under exclusive license to Springer Nature Switzerland AG 2021
J. S. Young, *Trauma Center Performance Improvement*,
https://doi.org/10.1007/978-3-030-71048-4_1

Definitions of Process Improvement and Patient Safety

There used to be clear delineations between performance improvement and patient safety; however, these two merged concepts in the past decade. Traditionally performance improvement and process improvement came from industry, especially the lean Toyota process and "efficiency experts." This personnel looked at manufacturing processes, attempted to remove waste, and improved efficiency while improving the end product quality. Patient safety primarily concerned itself with patient falls, medication errors, wrong-site surgery, etc. The American College of surgeons merges these two concepts into PIPS (performance improvement and patient safety) to encompass the process of examining and improving care delivery.

Examining traditional patient safety events is still part of performance improvement; however, all hospitals have patient safety departments that look at these events for their entire clinical enterprise. The trauma program may be asked to participate in these examinations, but the hospital PI program usually initiates them. Hospitals also spend a great deal of money and effort on performance improvement, primarily since mortality focuses on the joint commission. These PI efforts mirror those seen in trauma programs. The best programs transfer information between the trauma program in the hospital PI program, enhancing both processes.

What Is "Ego-Based" Medicine?

Surgeons are known for being aggressive, self-confident, and resistant to change. Trauma surgeons have many of these characteristics and have been indoctrinated to the critical need for self-examination and improvement. Every trauma program will run into "ego-based" medicine, especially in consultants. As we will discuss later, the corrective action for these problems is to bring these surgeons into the fold to see that the process is not punitive and is not criticizing their care but looking for a pathway for decreased variability in improved outcomes. There may still be surgeons who rebel against these efforts and often poison PI programs' success.

Evidence-based medicine can be an antidote for ego-based medicine. The trauma PI program's leadership must use scientific evidence as much as possible to support their analysis and corrective actions. As we know, only about 50% of current medical practice (or less) is supported by some level of scientific evidence. For these issues, the consensus is the antidote for ego-based medicine. Consensus requires acknowledging the problem, the willingness to listen to other people's opinions, and a desire to subvert one's ego to create a product that will benefit the patient.

Dealing with obstinate surgeons can be one of the most challenging jobs for a trauma medical director. It is challenging when the surgeons are in positions of authority in their departments. There are many strategies for dealing with these problems, and this book will illustrate several of them. Still, every trauma medical director must be ready for the fact that they will not achieve consensus in all areas. In those cases, it is crucial to thoroughly audit and analyze cases with adverse outcomes that could have been ameliorated by corrective action. By presenting these cases in group forums, resistance can sometimes be overcome or pushed to the background.

Science of Safety

There is considerable science around patient safety and performance improvement, and I learned a great deal from reading these investigators' works. James Reason's book *Human Error* is a classic description of the science of human error, scientific studies that have been performed, the types of error, and assessing the risk of critical error [2]. I also recommend the work of Gary Klein and Beth Crandall [3, 4].

Many other important leaders in the science of safety include W. Edwards Deming, A. Donabedian, Atul Gawande, among others. I feel that reading these authors has improved the scope of my knowledge of performance improvement, and I recommend them to all of you.

Most, if not all, PI efforts require data, but that is both a blessing and a curse. We learned that as regulatory agencies placed rewards and punishments on performance that any metric with sufficient importance can be "gamed." This is a critical problem because the gaming of metrics does not improve care. It also gives the program a false sense of security that their care is optimal and does not require improvement. So while metrics are necessary to most PI efforts, they are not an end in themselves.

Measuring too many processes in the trauma center can also be detrimental. Leaders must realize that two granular measurements lead to busywork and inefficient priorities. I mean that every program is limited in the amount of personnel they can employ. Suppose this personnel spends a great deal of their time merely collecting data, auditing charts to populate metrics that do not directly impact clinical outcomes. In that case, they will not have enough time left to perform performance improvement on those factors that do influence outcome.

Trauma programs are fortunate in that they are required to have a trauma registry. There are national standards for the components of a registry record, and there are also standards for the training and continuous education of the registrars. This means that quite often, the trauma registry in a trauma center is the most accurate source of data for trauma patients. The trauma quality improvement program (TQ IP) administered by the American College of surgeons allows trauma centers to benchmark their care against other similar centers nationwide. External benchmarking is essential in that without it, and a center can be satisfied with their performance and be ignorant that they are performing far below their peers. However, as I said before, when punishment or reward is based on metrics, you need to be very careful that the performance has not been gamed by data manipulation. A clear example of this is the fact that in many benchmarking systems, if the patient is formally transferred to a hospice program before death, that patient's death does not impact the hospital's benchmarking (the patient has been discharged to alive and dies in the hospice). These kinds of manipulations can seriously affect the quality of analysis in the program.

Studies have demonstrated that participation in surgical outcomes programs alone does not improve care [5, 6]. This further indicates that the use of metrics alone and the constant querying of databases do not in and of themselves constitute performance improvement.

Differentiating PI from the Discussion and Peer Review

The classic morbidity and mortality conference in surgery departments is a perfect example of peer review. Cases are presented and critiqued by experts in the field and colleagues, hopefully in a collegial environment. However, morbidity and mortality conferences tend to focus on physician decisions and technical issues rather than creating processes that decrease variability and improve outcomes. The program must be careful to differentiate discussion and peer review for performance improvement. The way to know that your discussion and peer review is performance improvement is that something is created at the end of the discussion that can be used as a corrective action, can be implemented, and audited. On the other side of this coin is that it is essential that the trauma program not undertake PI activities in a vacuum. Some PI programs focus exclusively on the trauma program manager and trauma medical director. These two individuals choose cases, analyze causes, and develop corrective actions often without input from the frontline providers and the clinical specialists. While this method is certainly possible to improve care, participation in PI activities by frontline personnel and clinicians is critical to buy-in and cooperation. Corrective actions imposed on clinicians without their input often fail or succeed for a short period and fade. It can be challenging for trauma programs to gain consensus and solicit opinions from a wide range of clinicians. Indeed, it is not necessary to involve everyone in the process. Still, nursing leaders, respiratory therapy leads, specialty physicians, and core trauma surgeons must have a say in the process.

References

1. Kohn LT, Corrigan JM, Donaldson MS, editors. To err is human: building a safer health system. Washington, D.C.: National Academy Press; 2000.
2. Reason J. Human error. New York: Cambridge University Press; 1990.
3. Klein G. Sources of power: how people make decisions. Cambridge, MA: MIT Press; 1999.
4. Crandall B, Klein GA, Hoffman RR. Working minds: a practitioners guide to cognitive task analysis. Cambridge, MA: A Bradford Book; 2006.
5. Etzioni DA, Wasif N, Dueck AC, Cima RR, Hohmann SF, Naessens JM, et al. Association of hospital participation in a surgical outcomes monitoring program with inpatient complications and mortality. JAMA. 2015;313(5):505–11.
6. Osborne NH, Nicholas LH, Ryan AM, Thumma JR, Dimick JB. Association of hospital participation in a quality reporting program with surgical outcomes and expenditures for Medicare beneficiaries. JAMA. 2015;313(5):496–504.

Chapter 2
Philosophy of PI

In this chapter, we discuss the philosophy of performance improvement. A proper philosophical belief in the importance of performance improvement in its ability to consistently improve the care provided to patients is critical to an effective PI program. There are many issues that can poison the effectiveness of the program, and we will discuss them.

Before we begin the discussion, I want to focus on one very important philosophical concept of performance improvement. It is that you must emphasize the positive when bringing the negative to light. In my own program, we just went through reawakening where every time someone from the trauma program contacted a clinician, he was to tell them that they did something wrong. No matter how you couch these discussions, consistently being looked at as the people that come tell you that something did not go right can lead to avoidance, hostility, and an overall depressive outlook toward the trauma program.

It is vitally important that the trauma program emphasizes the positive parts of trauma care in that institution. If you have no positive findings in your trauma center, then you should not fabricate positivity. However, in any center, positive processes can be identified and advertised. Even in the lowest-performing center, the trauma program can still celebrate the fact that a wide variety of clinicians are devoting a significant amount of time and effort to ensure that they provide as good care as possible to people having the worst days of their lives. Now it is the rarest center that cannot find some positive things to say. But even in centers that are high-performing, the trauma program can fall into the trap of only looking at metrics where they are performing poorly and only discussing deaths and adverse events. I can guarantee you that in a program that has a high-functioning performance improvement system, there are a lot of positives. A high-functioning PI system leads to positive outcomes, and if you do not see that, you are not looking for the right things. And if trauma care is a constantly negative and depressive act, then your hospital should reconsider being a trauma center and should consider having patients go to a center that can provide the care that is necessary.

J. S. Young, *Trauma Center Performance Improvement*,
https://doi.org/10.1007/978-3-030-71048-4_2

However, extremely low-performing trauma centers are not common. In fact, as a site reviewer, centers usually self-select themselves and are insightful enough to know that their trauma center is nonfunctional and usually will not proceed to ask for verification. The vast majority of other centers are doing a lot of things right and, in fact, are doing most things right. In high-performing centers, common mistakes are extremely uncommon. Performance improvement activities focus on gray areas within protocols and guidelines, situations where calm and cool reflection are not possible, leading to substandard decision-making, and an extremely critical mindset toward patients who do not survive. When my partner arrived, I had been running my PI program for about 10 years, and we had settled into what I would now see as complacency. When he stepped into the program, and I gave him PI is the primary role, he immediately started stirring things up. Processes that we had glossed over were now held up for scrutiny. This naturally caused some friction and negative feelings. Luckily during this time, we received reports of national benchmarking that showed that we were performing at a very high level. Thus, I would always advertise positive "press" along with whatever critiques that we meted out. Having been a coach for several sports, it is well known in that location that you must sandwich negative comments between positive comments. Constant negativity turns people off. Even in a case where things go badly, you should be able to go and find those aspects of the process that worked and couch your PI activities within a framework of encouragement and positivity.

Avoiding Bias and Ageism

In immature PI programs, you will often find bias against elderly patients' survival and against the survival of multiple-injured patients with hypovolemic shock. In many cases, this is unavoidable because these programs are not aware that patients at the extremes of age and at the extremes of injury can be saved and return to their families for years of quality life. If you have an 85-year-old patient with bilateral femur fractures and a pneumothorax, and in your experience, no patient this elderly and with this many injuries survives, then chances are that you cannot look at the processes in this case carefully, and you will merely determine the case is an unexpected death without opportunity for improvement.

When you encounter a 20-year-old patient who was found with the Glasgow coma score of five at the scene, has aspirated, and presents the emergency department with oxygen saturations of 80%, failed airway attempts, bilateral thoracic injuries, cervical spine fractures, pelvic fracture, and multiple additional orthopedic injuries along with hypotension, you will view this patient as unsurvivable. This is why it is critical for at least the leader of the trauma center to have spent a significant portion of time in a high-performing level I or level II center in order to see that both of these patients can survive and if care is provided in an optimal manner, will survive. However, if the clinicians in the trauma center have never encountered survival in these patients, it is difficult for them to properly analyze these cases for opportunities for improvement.

Therefore it is critical that every case be viewed initially as a unexpected mortality, and the process is to convince yourself that it is an expected mortality rather than starting with the idea that it is an expected mortality and convince yourself that it is unexpected. By doing the former, you will bring critical analysis to every adverse event and death regardless of the patient's age, physiologic status, and degree of injury.

This can be extremely difficult in centers where trauma surgeons, emergency physicians, and specialty liaisons do not have experience in high-performing trauma centers. These clinicians will push back against the trauma program's efforts to define certain deaths as unexpected, thus making it very difficult to carry out an effective PI process. For this reason, the American College of surgeons requires that the trauma medical director in a level I or II trauma center must have experience in a verified trauma center.

Triage of Issues

Not All PI Issues Are Created Equal.

Performance improvement issues can range from the trivial to the extremely serious. An example of a trivial issue could be the inability to find a certain piece of equipment that was not critical to the patient's outcome, and interpersonal interaction that was not optimal, or a simple medical record documentation problem that did not contribute to an adverse outcome. Serious PI issues include those that create harm for the patient or possibly death. These issues can include misdiagnosis, errors of commission, errors of omission, failure to rescue, misinterpretation of vital signs and diagnostic data, delays in treatment, delays and referral, delays, and transfer. No PI program has the ability to tackle every issue at the same time. The best PI programs create processes that allow them to handle most issues efficiently. The American College of surgeons expects that those issues that cause harm or death should be addressed immediately and aggressively. But even trivial issues, if repeated and centered on the same provider, can affect the performance of the trauma center, and you need to be addressed. In addition, some trivial issues could point to larger problems such as practitioner indifference, poor interpersonal interactions, or laziness.

It is the job of the trauma program manager or his/her designee to perform the initial triage of PI issues. After an issue is reported or is observed, they will try to gather real-time information about the problem from the people who witnessed or participated in the care of the patient. It is important to gather information quickly because personal observations tend to fade with time and if too much time elapses, you will be unable to reconstruct what actually happened. This may cause you to overreact or underreact to certain situations. Quite often, in the mature PI program, issues that appear to be serious are found to be overblown once an investigation is performed. And conversely, issues that seemed minor can sometimes be found to be serious after discussions with care providers and review of practitioner performance.

In general, patient death should have the highest priority for PI effort. The PI program should have a system where they are rapidly informed that a trauma patient has died and a process by which information is gathered about this patient rapidly and accurately. In our own program, our trauma PI coordinator often rounds in the ICU, so they are aware of patients that have died the night before or who may die that day, thus providing almost real-time information. Many hospitals have a daily huddle where serious events from the previous 24 hours are discussed among the caregivers. If such a system exists, then it is important that the PI lead person try to attend this huddle, or at least speak to someone who was at the hospital so they can gather information about the events that surrounded the patient's death. Once the initial information is gathered, then the PI lead and the physician PI lead should discuss the case and determine whether immediate analysis and corrective action are warranted. This would be warranted in the case where there was a high likelihood that a PI problem might recur and, if it did recur, cause patient harm. We will provide examples of this in the case studies at the end of this book.

Following death should be adverse events. Adverse events could be more difficult to collect, and the definition of what constitutes an adverse event varies among departments, programs, and institutions. An adverse event is generally considered to be an occurrence that adversely affects the patient's outcome. This can include many of the events that I described above, the only difference being that the patient survived. Also, remember that adverse events can occur in patients that do die days or weeks prior to their actual demise. Trauma patients will die, so it is impossible to have zero mortality, but it is possible to decrease the rate of adverse events through vigorous PI activities. The joint commission has recommendations for adverse event monitoring, and Medicare mandates recording and intervention for issues such as catheter-associated urinary tract infection, central line-associated bloodstream infection, healthcare-associated pressure ulcers, among other events. Since these events are also evaluated by the hospital performance improvement program, it is one of the issues why there needs to be close cooperation between the trauma program and the hospital quality program, so that parallel redundant effort does not occur. In addition, the hospital PI program may have corrective actions that will directly benefit trauma patients and vice versa, so spreading positive corrective actions requires information transfer between the trauma program in the hospital quality program. Adverse events are investigated in a similar manner to mortality; however, the time between occurrence and reporting for adverse events tends to be far longer than for mortality. There are various reasons for this, an important one being the discovery of the event and using a proper definition to classify an event. Many different systems have different definitions of adverse events, including TQIP, the joint commission, Medicare, etc. The trauma program should use trauma-related definitions of adverse events in order to provide consistency in the benchmarking of trauma centers. If every trauma center will have their own definition of urinary tract infection, then the aggregate data on urinary tract infections would be meaningless. This is where your trauma registrar becomes important because it is vital for them to use the proper definition when classifying an adverse event for entry into the registry. We have found in our own institution that we had strayed from the TQIP definitions, and thus our classification of adverse events had become inaccurate.

Below death and adverse events constitute many of the processes that occur every hour of every day in a trauma center. These include protocols and guidelines for the evaluation and treatment of injuries, guidelines for radiological evaluation, communication among caregivers, interpersonal interactions, equipment availability, operating room readiness, blood bank performance, and many other issues. In many cases, programs create "projects" that are long term in nature (sometimes as long as a year) to gather large amounts of information about an issue, create a task force to examine performance and provide recommendations for improvement, use this task force and the liaisons to implement a new process, and audit the new process. For instance, treatment of splenic injury, prevention of ventilator-associated pneumonia, and indications for MRI and spine injury are all appropriate issues for a "project." The reason why these issues are often aggregated into a greater effort is that they usually cannot be solved quickly and require input from thought leaders and content experts in specific areas, and they often require the creation of new guidelines that mandate review of the current evidence in the literature as well as gathering expert opinion.

Suboptimal interpersonal interactions are often covered by hospital bylaws, and a disciplinary process for practitioner misbehavior is usually hardwired. It can often be the job of the trauma program to report misbehavior up through the hospital chain of command. The trauma director would have little ability to discipline nurses, doctors, or any other healthcare providers that work with patients. Therefore, they must go through the personnel's chain of command to affect a change of behavior.

Frequent Versus Rare, Significant Harm Versus Trivial Harm

Triage of issues also depends on the rubric that ranks issues as to whether it is a rare event, a common event, can cause significant harm, or will cause trivial harm. The highest-ranked events are those that can cause significant harm and can occur frequently. The lowest-ranked events are those that are rare and cause trivial harm. Most issues lie somewhere in the middle. But this rubric does provide the program some guidance as to the triage of issues.

Beneficence All professionals have the foundational moral imperative of doing right. At the core of any trauma, the program is beneficent. This is the concept that all professionals have the fundamental moral imperative of doing right and avoiding harm. It is important to remember this concept when performing trauma PI.

This concept is exemplified by how the trauma program uses projects and pursues optimization of processes. It is impossible to deliver perfect clinical care. There will always be components of the care process that can be improved. The trauma program must prioritize their efforts on those aspects of the process of care that can determine morbidity and mortality for the patient. Sometimes this is not simple, and that there is no evidence for most of what we do in clinical medicine. Most clinical medicine is based on experience and expert opinion in trauma; especially, there are few randomized clinical trials to guide care. Hence, it is essential that the trauma program build consensus and avoid conflict unless it is absolutely necessary. Conflict breeds dissent, and dissent poisons the optimization of processes. It is impossible in many cases to get all physicians to agree to a plan of action, but by creating a consensus, the majority of clinicians can provide pressure on the outliers to conform. With regard to beneficence, it is vital for the trauma program to avoid actions that primarily benefit the clinician and not the patient. As an experienced reviewer for the American College of surgeons, I have often seen in level II and level III centers that processes are adapted to the following: decrease the need for the trauma surgeon to come in from home, lessen the chance that a face-to-face interaction in the middle of the night is necessary, and in general, put the comfort of the clinician above the outcome of the patient. To be honest most centers that do this occasionally do not really realize they are doing it. They feel they are merely fairly adapting their processes to the needs of their physicians. However, it is vital for the program to step back and look at these decisions from the standpoint of the patient. Does the patient benefit from creating a system where activations are downgraded to avoid having the trauma surgeon drive-in? This also applies to the interventional radiologist, the anesthesiologist, the orthopedist, the neurosurgeon, and all other specialties. It is extremely common in nonacademic centers to be gracious in allowing the trauma surgeon or specialist to remain at home. This does not necessarily mean care is inferior in the centers; it merely recognizes that with dozens of residents from the PGY one to PGY six level in the hospital at all times, it is far easier to bring some specialty knowledge and skill to the bedside and academic centers. However, if the hospital wants to hold itself out as being able to care for all manner of trauma patients, it is hard to justify that there are different requirements for in-person response between a level I, level II, or a level III center. It is difficult in many cases to enforce some of these rules because, as I said before, there is not a great deal of evidence showing that attending presence or subspecialty attending presence truly benefits outcome in the vast majority of cases. As a member of the verification review committee for many years, I have seen the committee tries hard as it can to balance optimal care versus unnecessarily burdening surgeons that are already extremely busy. But my comment is, "not every hospital needs to be a trauma center." And if you cannot organize your trauma center such that it is providing what is generally accepted to be the optimal care of the injured patient, then I believe you should consider not being a trauma center and not holding yourself out as a place that is providing state-of-the-art care for injured patients.

Another way of looking at this is ego-based medicine versus evidence-based medicine. I have seen repeatedly where surgeons will say, "I've never needed to be at the bedside for this," or "in my experience I dont need to be there…" to justify staying in bed. Not only is this used to justify staying at home, it is often used to justify minimalist attitudes toward injury. It is very difficult in retrospect to dissect whether a patient with a severe head injury who had an intracranial mass lesion that could be treated surgically was mismanaged by nonoperative care. But at the very least, in these cases, if the patient has an indication for operative management and a nonoperative course chosen, the fact that the neurosurgeon directly examined the patient and gathered their own findings and made a learned decision can be much more easily justified in making that decision over the phone. This is why being a trauma surgeon or specialist in a trauma center requires tremendous commitment. In this day and age, with most surgeons providing very little operating room care for injured patients (except the orthopedist), it is even harder to justify the extra time and effort on the part of specialist in trauma surgeons to provide care that will likely be poorly reimbursed and will only require observation and critical care. It is imperative that the trauma program, through the trauma director, cheerleading the effort and attitudes required to get yourself out of bed in the middle of the night and make the right decisions to optimize the outcome of the patient.

Finally, in difficult cases, there should be a discussion. Many trauma directors get into trouble when they are viewed as dictators making decisions in their office with the door closed. It is vital for effective PI that the trauma medical director and program manager foster relationships with key clinicians and administrators such that they can seek their advice in difficult situations and get their support when change is necessary.

Chapter 3
PI Techniques and Tools

In this chapter, we discuss the tools and techniques commonly used to improve care. I could put hundreds of references in this chapter, but I believe that is a waste of yours and my time. It is straightforward to look up the background of these techniques online and buy books to understand the concepts. Instead, I would look at the broad issues involved in each of these tools and techniques to help you choose which ones would be optimal for your situation. I will provide references for the materials I used to learn these systems, but they are in no way complete. There are hundreds of books on these systems.

All of these tools share some common threads. They involve finding a problem, analyzing the problem, developing an action plan, and carrying out that action plan. All of these different techniques revolve around those four key processes.

PDSA

Deming [1] introduced the PDCA and PDSA cycles. We will talk about the PDSA since it is the one that I am most familiar with. PDSA stands for plan, do, study, act. It is also known as plan, do, check, and act. I think that this technique is the easiest to understand, although it does not include the hard work needed to ensure that you pick up on adverse events or suboptimal processes.

However, PDSA does help you organize the flow of PI activities. For a simple example, let us say you miss a spleen injury, admitted the patient to the floor, and the patient dies hemorrhagic shock. The planning part of this problem is fairly easy; you do not want people to die of injuries that you could diagnose and treat. And your goal or objective is to not miss any life-threatening injuries. They do part of this process and would include figuring out what had gone wrong and figuring out how to prevent it from happening again in the future (I am not going to go into a detailed description of how to handle this problem now as we will discuss these

J. S. Young, *Trauma Center Performance Improvement*,
https://doi.org/10.1007/978-3-030-71048-4_3

issues in the case review chapters). The check or study part of the cycle would be to determine whether the changes that you put in place during the do phase are actually being followed and are having the desired result. In the active phase, you would be taking everything you learned and adjusted as needed to reevaluate the process and determine if you should proceed with the plan that you initiate in the do phase or go back and re-examine the problem and come up with a new action plan.

The PDSA system is somewhat simplistic and leaves out a fair amount of steps. The other PI techniques we will discuss help the PI professional find, examine, and correct problems a little bit more easily. However, the more complex the tool is, the more time you need to spend learning it and implementing it. PDSA is fairly simple, easy to understand, and easy to follow. However, Deming created this for manufacturing processes primarily, and his translation of clinical medicine is not perfect.

Brent James and Intermountain Health [2]

About 20 years ago, I traveled to Salt Lake City, Utah, to take the course in performance improvement provided by Intermountain healthcare and directed by Dr. Brent James. I would consider Brent James to be my intellectual mentor in performance improvement. I do not work with him directly, and we do not often communicate; however, what I was taught 20 years ago I still use every day.

Dr. James basically teaches that you should try to keep performance improvement simple and straightforward. First, you find a problem, then you try to figure out what went wrong, then try to figure out a way to correct it, and then you correct it, and then you see if it was fixed. He also stresses that complex data collection systems and complex auditing systems are not necessary. A simple piece of paper or simple spreadsheet is all that is needed to keep track of a problem, keep track of the interventions, and determine if the problem was fixed. Dr. James still teaches this course in Utah, and I would encourage people in medicine who are interested in becoming PI professionals to travel there and take this course.

Six Sigma [3]

Six Sigma is one of the complex PI tools available today. Almost everyone reading this book is probably heard of Six Sigma and knows that it involves an adaptation of belts that are given out to define advancement in the martial arts. There are green belts, black belts, and master black belts. I was a Greenbelt and went through the Six Sigma training program. However, I have truly found the Six Sigma did not provide that much more useful information than I gathered from Dr. James. The core of Six Sigma is DMAIC, which stands for define, measure, analyze, improve, check, or control. As you can see, this parallels all of the tools that I have already provided. Six Sigma does provide some interesting techniques to explain how to overcome resistance and gain consensus. But you will learn as you make performance improvement that much of overcoming resistance and gaining consensus depends on the person who is controlling the process. If you are dictatorial, chances are resistance will merely be pushed underground. If you do not listen to multiple viewpoints, you will never gain consensus, and your PI process will fail. Six Sigma does provide more eloquent ways of describing this, but these are the basics.

Lean [4]

The Lean system is a derivation of a system created by the Toyota Motor Company to improve the output and quality of their product. It grew from manufacturing plants, and some of its core ideals are that you must go to the front line to actually see how processes are implemented, you should gather information quickly after events, you should have a system where anyone can "stop the line" (meaning that you listen to the frontline caregivers since they are the ones that know the process most intimately).

The Lean system uses the "A3" as the basic tool for improvement. The A3 is the designation for a certain type of printer paper that is 11x17 that was used by Toyota engineers to document and plan improvement projects. There are hundreds of books written on the Lean system (and the Lean Six Sigma system), and I cannot do the system justice in a few pages.

Some positive aspects of the Lean system are the ways that it guides and focuses the improvement work. The process is divided into problem statement (what the issue is) or background, current condition, goal, root cause analysis, countermeasures, effect confirmation, and follow-up. This provides a more concrete framework than the simple PDSA, and there is examination and discussion of each step. For Lean coaches, there is little need for content expertise. They are trained in the system and use a variety of tools (the five why's, etc.) to help the PI coordinator to refine what the problem is (and restrict it to a reasonable scope), take the necessary time to define the current condition (through data analysis, survey, or direct observation), define where you want the process to be when finished, do a thorough root cause analysis (where the five why's are used), design countermeasures that are doable, and which do not worsen the problem by unnecessarily burdening the frontline worker with extra work and time requirements, thorough design of countermeasures, and a re-examination of the process and follow-up.

While many hospital based quality programs are using Lean, few PI programs use all the tools in the Lean program. Though I feel Lean has the best framework for PI activity, it is fairly technical, rigid, and often expensive in that coaches are necessary. Though this may only be my personal experience with it, the documentation is excessive, the number of meetings necessary is a problem for many, and the sponsors are often able to derail improvement by forcing the PI practitioners to refocus, restrict, or otherwise adapt their conclusions to ones that are less expensive.

But the Lean program does not need to be implemented in the way I observed, and no PI program needs to adopt a program in its entirety. Lean provides many excellent tools and concepts, and PI programs should take what they like and discard the rest if it serves their purposes well.

TOPIC [5]

TOPIC is the PI system taught by the Society for Trauma Nursing and is the most common system I have observed in US trauma centers. The course is put on regularly, and I encourage all TPMs, TMDs, and PI coordinators to attend the course or work with a program that has implemented its concepts.

I will not reiterate the TOPIC program here, but it basically includes tools from many systems and an escalation rubric that helps programs properly triage and address minor and major issues. I encourage you to find out more about TOPIC since it is pretty much the standard system for trauma center PI.

There are many other systems and tools out there. What I want to reiterate is that no system or tool is perfect for every situation. PDSA does not provide sufficient tools to break down certain issues; Six Sigma and Lean are complex and require specific training and personnel. TOPIC is excellent but lacks some of the specific tools found in the other systems.

Our synthesis at UVA of these systems is as follows:

- Having a person who is devoted solely to PI activities or ensures that a defined and protected part of the TPM's duties are allocated to PI. In busy programs, it is virtually impossible for the TPM to carry the PI program and all their other responsibilities.
- Creating a system where all PI activities can be easily tracked. The system includes the issue, the responsible party, the outcomes of reviews, minutes from meetings, corrective action documents, loop closure documents, and the timeline.
- Having a "tactical" meeting each week that includes the core PI staff. In this meeting, cases from the past 7 days a reviewed, and urgent issues can be immediately elevated. In most trauma centers, the interval between monthly PI meetings is too long in many centers and have other meetings between their main peer review/PI meetings in order to begin the PI process around various issues.

While almost all centers have a "morning report" process where cases from the previous night are discussed and expectations for the coming day are outlined, ours, as well as others, have a weekly trauma conference whose attendees include nurse practitioners, physician assistants, trauma attendings, residents and medical students, pharmacists, and other personnel as needed. This conference is used as a critical dissemination tool of corrective action plans. It can also be used to present cases and gather opinions from a variety of personnel to bring a broad analysis. It is also an important venue for the attending of record in the treating residents and nurse practitioners to provide their input so that the PI program can have a better understanding of the facts and events that surrounded the PI issue.

No PI program that I have ever examined follows a distinct PI system to the letter. As I have outlined above, while each of the systems may have many positive attributes, each of them lacks some tools. As I have stated previously, Six Sigma provides excellent tools for breaking down an issue and taking the road to improvement, but this system is expensive in that it requires coaches (black belts) and extensive training, which many centers do not have the resources to implement. The Lean system also requires coaches, a multitude of meetings, and a very rigid system for issue analysis and intervention that many may find onerous. TOPIC provides trauma-relevant information, and as I stated, is probably overall the best system for a trauma center to use, but it still lacks some of the tools of the others.

I recommend that every trauma program manager in PI coordinator experience the topic course in that it is the gold standard for PI in US trauma centers. However, the site visitor will not penalize the center if it does not use TOPIC as long as their PI system identifies issues, analyzes them, gets broad input, develops pertinent corrective action plans, implements those plans, and follows up. In fact, many mature PI programs use none of these tools and yet do a fantastic job of creating optimal care.

Now that we have discussed some of the tools, trends, and fads that revolve around improving quality, let us talk about what are the major components that every performance improvement program must have. First, the program has to have a method suitable for identifying issues. This can be simple or complex or a combination of both: Simply a member of the trauma program or the trauma team goes through admissions and discharges from the previous evening and day and identifies those patients that were admitted with injuries either to the trauma service or to a specialty service. Usually, hospitals will provide a list of those patients have expired in the previous day in this list should be examined as well. Most experienced trauma registrars have developed a system that has multiple inputs to ensure that they do not miss any trauma admissions or any trauma discharges or death. Any of the more common trauma registry education programs will provide a framework for this.

As far as specific issues related to patient care, the trauma program must advertise to the entire health system that they are to be notified whenever someone has a concern about the treatment of the trauma patient or the conduct of somebody caring for trauma patients. While this could be part of an error or conduct reporting system integral to the health system, it can also simply involve an email to the trauma medical director or the trauma program manager. Also, many issues were identified simply by walking through the surgical ICU or meeting people in the hall. What is important is that these issues are properly triaged and addressed and are not allowed to fester.

No matter the type or process of issue identification, the program must have a consistent method for examining these issues in properly triaging them. For deaths, that is fairly straightforward, and that all deaths need to undergo TPM and TMD review. For clinical issues, this can be more difficult. Issues related to physician practice can be referred by the trauma medical director to the specialty liaisons, and issues related to nursing or other clinician practice can be referred to the appropriate nursing hierarchy. The key in these referrals is that there is a feedback loop where the trauma program should know that the issue has been addressed and the solution has been put in place.

Some issues require a more involved PI process. These are issues that I described previously that either can represent significant harm to a single patient or multiple patients or can present moderate harm to a large number of patients or even trivial harm to a large number of patients. These issues usually require a concerted effort on the part of the trauma PI program to examine the root causes and develop a corrective action plan. This will usually involve several weeks of work in several meetings. The usual process is that the trauma program manager or PI coordinator takes the issue and gathers more specific information while it is still fresh in the minds of the clinicians. They then take this information and discuss it with the trauma program manager and the trauma medical director to determine the next course of action. I want to stress at this point that the program must have a low threshold for escalating issues to the stage of corrective action. One of the red flags for site visit inspections is when a large number of issues that are entered into the trauma program PI process are disposed of with little or no investigation and no attempt at corrective action. Do not confuse what I am saying in that not every small issue requires a PI project, but when issues impacted the care of the patient, almost invariably it requires some documentation and some discussion within the trauma PI core personnel and should also warrant some documentation in the PI records that can demonstrate to the site visit team that you took a thorough look at the issue and determine that either it was a rare event or that the effects on patient care were so trivial that a complex corrective action plan would only make the process more complicated and possibly worse. You can certainly dispose of issues in this way, and every program does, but you need to have a rationale for why he disposed of it. That rationale cannot be that it will be too hard to fix. "Things happen" is not a root cause that can be used often.

The program, once it is identified as issues that need to be elevated, needs to have a fairly prescribed process of how it examines the issues, properly identifies root causes, develops countermeasures, and then develops a corrective action plan. Many programs have wonderful corrective action plans that do not get implemented or get implemented in a haphazard manner. Good mature PI programs have excellent follow-through on corrective action plans either through defined education programs; creation of guidelines, conferences, and dissemination of information; and a robust auditing process to ensure that the corrective action plan actually alleviated the problem.

So the process of identification, analysis, triage, investigation, corrective action plan creation, dissemination, and follow-up is the key technique that every PI program must use.

References

1. Deming WE. Out of the crisis. Cambridge, MA: MIT Press; 1986. p. 88.
2. Brent James MD (https://intermountainhealthcare.org/blogs/authors/brent-james-md/).
3. Anbari FT. Six sigma method and its applications in project management, proceedings of the Project Management Institute annual seminars and symposium [CD], San Antonio, Texas. Oct 3–10. Project Management Institute, Newtown Square, PA. 2002.
4. Holweg M. The genealogy of lean production. J Oper Manag. 2007;25:420–37. https://doi.org/10.1016/j.jom.2006.04.001.
5. Trauma Outcome and Performent Improvement Course, Society for Trauma Nurses TOPIC (https://www.traumanurses.org/topic).

Chapter 4
Program Personnel and Regulatory Requirements

Virtually every trauma center in the United States has to follow a set of guidelines or regulations. Some centers are regulated by the state where they reside, the American College of Surgeons committee verifies others on trauma, and others have to fulfill requirements set forth by both their state and the ACS. ACS verification requirements are detailed in the "optimal resources for the care of the injured patient" created by the ACS COT and is regularly updated. This document is created by teams of trauma surgeons and trauma program managers who manage ACS-verified trauma centers. The content of this book and the conduct of the ACS verification program are controlled by the verification review committee, which is a subcommittee of the committee on trauma. The executive committee of the committee on trauma approves all changes to the program.

I have been a member of the verification review committee for over 16 years. I have been involved in drafting criteria, writing chapters of the optimal resources document, and setting standards for site visitors. Thus, I have a pretty thorough knowledge of this process. Initially, when the optimal resources document was created, there was very little scientific data to support many of the criteria. Even now, high-quality data is rare for many of the requirements in the document. As the years have gone by, the COT has adopted criteria to fit the current evidence. But still, a large number of the criteria are based on expert opinion, committee consensus, and experience. The committee on trauma expends great effort to solicit opinions from verified trauma centers as to the effectiveness of criteria if this information is taken into account when revisions are made.

Performance improvement deficiencies are the most common critical deficiencies identified during site visits. However, this is improved over the years as various organizations have provided education to trauma program managers and medical directors. Also, the committee on trauma encourages young programs to partner

© The Author(s), under exclusive license to Springer Nature Switzerland AG 2021   23
J. S. Young, *Trauma Center Performance Improvement*,
https://doi.org/10.1007/978-3-030-71048-4_4

with more mature trauma centers to learn from their PI programs. I encourage any hospital that is starting its trauma center journey to find a nearby ACS-verified center to visit, ask questions of, and even emulate when necessary. There is no reason to reinvent the wheel when it comes to performance improvement. Though each hospital may have distinct characteristics that need to be taken into account, if you take care of injured patients, the general processes of identification, analysis, identification of root causes, correction action plan creation, and implementation are common to all centers.

Leadership

The trauma medical director should be the leader of the PI program. The trauma program manager works with the trauma medical director to carry out the day-to-day operations of the program. Many mature trauma centers designate a second physician to be the associate director whose portfolio is performance improvement. And many centers hire a second nurse to supplement the trauma program manager and service the PI coordinator performance improvement in a daily, if not an hourly process. A center that carries out the processes of performance improvement only once a month when they have a scheduled meeting cannot possibly be effective. The monthly multidisciplinary performance improvement meeting or peer review meeting, as many programs call it, should be a meeting where the products of the PI process are presented for general discussion, consensus building, and approval of corrective action plans.

It is often the role of the associate trauma medical director in the PI coordinator to organize a weekly meeting to go over cases that may grow into PI issues. This meeting is also used to keep track of current corrective action plans, make adaptations as necessary, coordinate with liaisons, and ensure that progress moves forward and does not stall. Since the American College of Surgeons only requires the multidisciplinary PI meeting, many programs are confused about how to demonstrate the work that goes on in an additional weekly meeting. My recommendation is simply to add notes to charts or PI logs that reflect what is undertaken during their weekly meetings. You can also generate a separate set of minutes for this meeting; they can be integrated into the overall documentation of the PI program. We will talk more about meetings in a subsequent section.

Data Collection

Data collection is necessary for a PI program, but the PI program must be more than just data.

I have seen quite a few PI programs that feel that they are operating at the high end because they have a great number of charts and spreadsheets. Data is necessary in order to maintain situational awareness of your program, identify deaths, adverse events, and near misses, understand your nonsurgical admissions, emergency department dwell times, time to surgery in those patients that require emergency operations, and overall hospital and ICU length of stay. But just collecting this data and presenting it in some form do not constitute performance improvement. You can have megabytes of data, but if you do not analyze it and use it to optimize care, then it is of very little use.

The trauma registrar is the team member most associated with effective and efficient data collection. I will not go into how the registry works or how a trauma registrar can organize their activities because there are too many tools, courses, and literature out there to help the program. I will state that it is important for the trauma registrar to be integrated into the PI program. They must understand what issues are important to the trauma center leadership; they must be familiar with how the trauma center leisure once this data is presented and how often it wants it collected, and most importantly, the registry must be able to supply ad hoc reports as needed.

These ad hoc reports can be a very important part of the PI program. When we do site visits, we will always ask the registrar to do an ad hoc report to see first whether they are able to do it, second how accurate it is, and third how well they understand the variables in the registry to put them together to provide a new query. Every program must have a certain number of filters; however, you should have more than the minimum number of queries, and you should develop new queries as problems come up. You cannot possibly maintain data collection and analysis for hundreds of different questions, some will start to have a short half-life and then die, and others, such as deaths and adverse events, will persist throughout the life of your program. This book mostly concerns itself with case-based PI, but I will take some time here to discuss the usefulness of ad hoc queries.

In your PI meeting, you present a case where a patient with an intracranial mass lesion did not get to the operating room for 7 hours after the CT scan. While it is necessary to examine this case specifically, it would be a loss of an opportunity not to look back and look at the performances in the realm of emergency operations for intracranial mass lesions. A good registrar should be able to respond to the question relatively quickly (however, we know that without a specific field for intracranial pressure monitoring, determining the frequency of that procedure can be difficult). The query can be as simple as filtering for patients who underwent craniotomy in the first 24 hours and then reviewing these charts to understand the interval between diagnosis and surgery, or can be more complex by looking at a filter for epidural and subdural hematoma was and then looking at what percentage of those patients went to the operating room in the first 24 hours and then drilling down.

I feel it is important to cast these queries somewhat widely at the beginning. If you make a narrower query, simply by missing a diagnosis code or procedure code, you may not find all the data that you are looking for. In my experience, I have asked for very specific queries and have received numbers that do not make sense (such as querying for certain splenic laceration diagnosis codes to try to understand the spectrum of splenic lacerations and finding a low number because these codes are not used frequently). In a perfect world, we would have trauma registries with some artificial intelligence that could take a basic question and expanded in such a way to run multiple queries and identified the most accurate one. However, we are not at that stage, and registry queries still require a fair amount of hit or miss filtering.

At its most basic, a PI program must examine every death; therefore, the program must have an ability to identify patients that die no matter where they are in the hospital. For example, patients with isolated hip fractures may be admitted to medicine with an orthopedic consult. In some site visits, I have done, I have seen patients admitted to neurology, medicine, or pediatrics without any surgical consult that died, and these cases can often be the most difficult for the program to examine since the components of the trauma program have little to no involvement. The registrar has to have a foolproof system for identifying patients that have died in the previous 24 hours.

It is often more difficult to identify adverse events and near misses. Most hospitals have a safety reporting program, but this program may not be integrated into the trauma program and may have an entirely parallel pathway of identification, analysis, and corrective action. This is why the American College of Surgeons has begun to concentrate more heavily on examining the integration of the trauma PI program with the overall hospital quality program. It is important that the trauma PI program attend hospital quality meetings and that there is a back-and-forth flow of information concerning issues of interest. Often the trauma program manager and medical director need to spearhead this effort.

In summary, the trauma registry is the foundation for data collection in the trauma center, but there need to be other tendrils that extend through patient care units, the emergency department, and other units of the hospital to identify issues that may impact trauma patients. Hence, the trauma program manager, or PI coordinator, has to be able to integrate smoothly into many different quality programs in order to gather the data necessary to optimize care.

Meetings

The American College of Surgeons mandates a multidisciplinary PI meeting in a systems improvement meeting. Often these meetings are combined since the attendees overlap. Some programs have a separate peer review meeting where the physicians review clinical decision-making and clinical performance without nonphysicians in attendance. Often this is due to legal restrictions and estate concerning the discoverability of peer review. However, in most centers, monthly multidisciplinary PI meetings and systems improvement meetings are often held on the same day, one following the other.

There is a good deal of detail outlining the attendees for the multidisciplinary PI meeting. This includes the trauma program manager, trauma medical director, trauma PI coordinator, the trauma registrar, the trauma surgeons, the liaisons, representatives from the ED, radiology, operating room, laboratory, and often the managers of the key clinical care units taking care of injured patients. The trauma surgeons and the liaisons are required to attend 50% of these meetings on a yearly basis. Attendance should be clearly documented and available for site review teams, and it is often important that 12 months before your site visit, you evaluate the attendance of the mandatory members of the committee and ensure that those that may not have attended 50% know that they must do that and attend every meeting before the site visit. This is a simple task for the site reviewer to see that one of the core individuals did not attend 50% of the meetings in the previous 12 months, and this is a criteria deficiency. In the day and age of our current pandemic, I believe all of these meetings should have a virtual option, and there is virtually no excuse for a committee member to miss a virtual meeting. I also believe that virtual meetings provide a good method for interaction, presentation materials, and discussion. I believe going forward, most programs will have a combination of face-to-face and virtual meetings.

The agenda for the multidisciplinary PI meeting usually consists of the following:

- Review of open issues
- Presentation of deaths without opportunities for improvement (OFI)
- Detailed presentation of deaths with OFI
- Review of process and system issues
- Review of site visit preparation
- Review of open time for discussions

Many programs have very large agendas for the multidisciplinary PI meetings where the minutes extend to over a dozen pages. Your program manager can do whatever he feels is necessary to fulfill the requirements of the PI program. Be mindful that meetings over 2 hours and over ten agenda items begin to lose the crowd. You want your attendees to be engaged and enthusiastic about discussing ways to improve your program. Often these meetings are recorded and transcribed later. Minutes are necessary for the site visit team to review and for you to be aware of what has been discussed in the past, and to go back and confirm key points. While two dozen pages of minutes are excessive, one page is not sufficient. The minutes should include all aspects of the agenda, should include the slides that were presented to the committee, and should include a transcribed discussion of the opportunities for improvement in order to demonstrate to the site visit team cogent analysis and critical review. Some states restrict this sort of documentation due to the discoverability of peer review discussions. This is unfortunate in those trauma centers in the states that need to devise a way to demonstrate to the site visit team that they are carrying out effective PI activities. One way to do this is to aggregate issues into "projects" that are conglomerations of multiple patients and thus de-identified to the individual patient. Also, documentation of cases and discussion can have all private health information removed wherein it is often not necessary to know the patient's name for the case to proceed through the PI process. Cases can simply be numbered in these numbers, or registry designations can be used to follow the case through the process. This is burdensome, but in many states, the programs need to find an innovative solution to protect themselves and allow for vigorous peer review.

It is becoming more common for programs to have weekly meetings in addition to their monthly multidisciplinary PI meeting. Tackling problems once a month, especially in a program that depends on group consensus to move forward, often severely delays the identification of problems and implementation of corrective action plans. In our program, we have a weekly "tactical" meeting of the key members of the PI program, including the medical director assigned to performance improvement, the PI coordinator, the trauma registrar, and the trauma program manager. At this meeting, new cases are quickly discussed and triaged. If there are obstacles to improvement becoming evident, this meeting can be used to identify those obstacles in a more expeditious manner. Many programs also have a weekly case conference. In our facility, we provide food on a Friday afternoon meeting where all of the highest level activations, deaths, and major complications are presented in front of our trauma attendings, advanced practice personnel, and resident staff. Pharmacy and nursing unit management also attend this meeting. This is a great opportunity for discussion, to find out the real story behind the care of certain patients that is indecipherable from the medical record, and to build camaraderie among all members of the team. When a sensitive case is being presented, the leader of the program should chair the meeting to ensure that it does not become contentious.

Chapter 5
Program Setup

We have already covered the basics of the PI program structure. We will now go into some of the specifics of how you create situational awareness of your program and find opportunities for improvement.

What Is Reviewed?

Deaths

First and most importantly is the review of injured patients who die at your hospital. This ranges from multiple trauma patients to the elderly patient with an isolated hip fracture. As we already stated, it can be difficult, especially for patients not admitted to a surgical service, to identify all injured patients who die accurately. The registrar should work with the hospital to insure that the trauma program is expeditiously informed of deaths in trauma patients.

There are many ways to examine trauma deaths. I will outline the process at my trauma center, and the TOPIC course gives excellent guidance on this TOPIC. Registrars are informed of all patients who died in the hospital in the previous 24 hours by 9 AM the following morning; she then prioritizes the abstracting of these patients' charts immediately. Our hospital also uses a Lean system of performance improvement where a huddle takes place between the nurse manager, treating physician, bedside nurse, and any other clinicians involved with the patient immediately after death to identify opportunities for improvement and obtain information as close to real time as possible. Our PI coordinator is also informed of all deaths in the hospital in the previous 24 hours and will contact clinicians to gather information about the patient. Suppose these efforts identify a critical opportunity for improvement that may affect many other patients adversely. In that case, the PI coordinator immediately contacts the trauma program manager, trauma medical

© The Author(s), under exclusive license to Springer Nature Switzerland AG 2021
J. S. Young, *Trauma Center Performance Improvement*,
https://doi.org/10.1007/978-3-030-71048-4_5

director, and associate trauma medical director for PI to discuss the case and see if a rapid improvement process is necessary. This process entails immediately gathering the key players in the PI program, the hospital's quality program, and relevant services to discuss the case and the opportunity for improvement and see if immediate solutions can be put into effect. But these are rare instances in which we have only had probably half a dozen in 20 years, and most of these have surrounded equipment failures.

Suppose no immediate concerns are depending on the day of the week. In that case, the case is presented at our Friday "chicken" conference, which is a mini morbidity and mortality, highest level activation review, and teaching conference where all members of the trauma team, including nurse practitioners, attendings, residents, students, pharmacy, and anyone else interested attends. The chicken aspect of this conference is the food that we consistently provide. As we have stated earlier, we also have a tactical PI conference every Tuesday to review new PI cases and old PI cases that have stagnated or have had recent movement. Thus if the death occurs Saturday through Tuesday, it is discussed Tuesday; if it occurs Wednesday or Thursday or Friday, it is discussed Friday. The case is presented with the relative X-rays and laboratory results, and the chief resident will usually provide their insight into the patient's care. This presentation will begin with EMS activation and go through to the patient's demise. At this conference, we will solicit opinions on opportunities for improvement, and more often, the actual caregivers involved will be there to provide their insight. The Tuesday tactical PI conference is attended by the trauma PI coordinator, the trauma registrar, administrative assistant, trauma program manager, and associate trauma medical director. They will review the deaths and determine whether the death can be declared anticipated without opportunity for improvement and can be slated for presentation at the next multidisciplinary PI conference. If it is either unanticipated with OFI, anticipated with OFI, or unanticipated without OFI (which is a rare classification), then the normal PI process proceeds with a thorough write up of the entire case, further discussion, solicitation of opinions from liaisons, and then a formal multiple slide presentation at the MDPI conference. At this conference, we use a web-based voting system to query the attendees about their opinions concerning our analysis and the need for corrective action. The votes are recorded and are made part of the PI record. The PI process then proceeds to execute the corrective action plan, ensure that the new process is in place, and evaluate whether the OFI has been properly disposed of.

Audit Filters

Every program must have audit filters to monitor the care delivered in the trauma center. Mortality is the one mandatory audit filter, but the program should also create a variety of other filters that create situational awareness of the care being provided at their trauma center. These audit filters can revolve around routine daily processes (emergency department while time, ICU length of stay, hospital length of stay) or known complications such as ventilator-associated pneumonia, catheter-associated urinary tract infection, central line-associated bloodstream infections, healthcare-associated pressure ulcers, and unplanned return to the operating room. In addition, every program should monitor the activation of the massive transfusion protocol to ensure first that the protocol is being followed and second that is being called appropriately.

There were few audit filters that the American College of Surgeons site visit team would object to, and the programs have leeway in deciding on these filters. However, if, in the site visitor's opinion, the care appears to be consistently suboptimal, they would expect the trauma program to be vigorously and aggressively looking at the care they provide in identifying cases for improvement through carefully constructed audit filters that are regularly queried.

For instance, if the center identifies several head injury deaths associated with a delayed neurosurgical response, then the center should set an audit filter to review all patients admitted with the G CS of eight or less over at least a 6-month time span. They should bring in the neurosurgery liaison to discuss what the standard response should be to head-injured patients; if this response is consistently not occurring, they should provide direct and immediate feedback to the neurosurgeons who are not responding appropriately. In some cases, neurosurgeons need to be removed from the trauma panel because they simply cannot meet the standard set by the trauma medical director and the neurosurgery liaison. In academic centers, the problem may be with the neurosurgical residents, who are not properly communicating with their chief residents and attendings. Since these lower-level residents will undoubtedly be defensive, it is very important to put them in a no-blame environment so that you can learn what is going on. One of the easier ways to do this is to use the brain trauma foundation guidelines, work through these with the neurosurgical liaison to identify those guidelines that have the strongest evidence and that they wish to be implemented, educate all clinicians in the program as to the neurosurgery guidelines that are put in place for the trauma center including nurses and frontline staff. Once staff are educated, it becomes relatively simple for a trauma service clinician or nurse that sees a deviation from these guidelines to begin a discussion with the clinician about the deviation. To ensure the patient is getting optimal care.

Below is the list of audit filters that we use at the University of Virginia:

Averages:
- Hospital LOS, ICU LOS, injury severity score
- W Scores
- ISS and Deaths by ranges

PI Audits:
- Patients admitted to an ICU without a trauma activation
- Deaths that occur in the first 24 hours without a trauma activation
- Patients with ISS greater than or equal to 15 without a trauma activation
- Cribari matric [1] (over and undertriage for all patients and for prehospital patients)

Activations:
- Alpha attending presence in 15 minutes
- Activation upgrades
- Activation downgrades
- Beta alerts (I audit a percent, not 100%) attending note signed within 8 hours
- Gamma alerts (audit a percent not 100%) attending note signed within 24 hours

Other filters
- ED temps
- Percent readmissions
- Epidural / subdural / with a midline shift: Number of patients with neuro consult within 30 minutes

- Tetraplegia patients with neuro / ortho consult within 30 minutes
- Mangled extremity or vascular compromise with ortho consult within 30 minutes
- Hemodynamically unstable pelvic fractures with ortho consult within 30 minutes
- ED transfer out to acute care (burns)

Performance Measures and Benchmarking Tools

Even the most self-critical trauma program cannot reliably identify suboptimal performance in all aspects. It is necessary to look outside your program at the aggregate performance of similar trauma centers to determine whether you are above or below the median performance. The trauma quality improvement project (TQIP) is an outstanding program administered by the American College of Surgeons that gathers extensive data on trauma admissions from all levels of trauma centers throughout the United States. It now has millions of patients in the database and an oversight committee staffed by extremely bright and capable trauma surgeons, registrars, and program managers that adapt the program as needed to provide optimal tools for performance improvement.

There are usually two reports per year from TQIP. In these reports, risk-adjusted benchmarking is provided for the following:

- Mortality
- Major complications
- Major complications including death
- Specific complications

    – Acute kidney injury
    – Ventilator-associated pneumonia
    – Pulmonary embolism
    – Surgical site infection
    – Unplanned admission to the ICU
    – Unplanned return to the OR
    – Catheter-associated UTI

- Resource utilization
- Comorbid conditions
- Discharge disposition
- Processes of care

It is impossible for a program to audit and monitor every process that may impact the patient's outcome. Obviously, mortality is the most important filter, and then there are filters that are required by regulatory agencies. The program should have the flexibility to choose other items to audit. In this way, the PI program stays fresh, looks at different problems during the year, devises innovative solutions, and shows the rest of the hospital that it is constantly trying to improve care.

The setup of the trauma PI program should promote efficiency, nimbleness, and effectiveness. To meet these goals, it must be able to act quickly and with purpose. It also must take a wide-angle look at the overall performance of the trauma center to ensure that trauma care is consistently improving.

There are many factors that can affect the performance of a trauma center that is outside the purview of the trauma center management. For instance, senior attendings can retire or be moved to other trauma centers, key nursing positions can turn over, and the hospital may decide that it is not going to put adequate resources behind the care of injured patients. Therefore, it is so vital for the trauma program director or trauma program manager to fight for adequate resources to carry out their mission. This means a strong registry and registrar, adequate administrative staff to organize meetings and documentation, sufficient time for the trauma program manager to execute PI activities or to hire a PI coordinator, and to adequately compensate the trauma medical director for the time that he or she must spend overseeing the performance of the trauma program. The American College of Surgeons verification program does provide a cudgel that can allow trauma centers to influence hospital administration to provide adequate resources. There are minimum requirements for program staff by the ACS, and the staff must be present, or the center will not be verified. However, once adequate resources are in place, they need to be used optimally. To do this, the program must have an efficient method for identifying problems, performing analysis, creating corrective action plans, implementing them, and auditing.

Reference

1. Harrell KN, Spain SJ, Whiteaker KA, Poulson JL, Barker DE. Modified need for trauma intervention criteria reduces cribari trauma overtriage rate. J Trauma Nurs. 2020;27(4):195–9.

Chapter 6
Trauma Registries and Other Data Sources

This will be a short chapter outlining some information about trauma registries and the role in the performance improvement process. There are many excellent resources available, which I will cite at the end of this chapter and that will do a much better job at explaining registry functions than I can. I will focus on some of the basics and how the registry should be used to enhance the performance improvement process.

Purpose of the Registry

The presence of a trauma registry is what separates trauma center care from most other endeavors in medicine. While cancer registries and other registries (such as transplant registries) may exist, many of them are intended for long-term examination of outcomes and demographics and not to be used as a tool for real-time performance improvement. Many people will state that the trauma registry does not usually function in real time, and in many centers, an event will occur, registry abstraction will occur, and the PI investigation will begin all within a short period of time.

Registry operations and quality control are vital for obtaining accurate data about your patient population. Having sufficient numbers of registrars who can get to charts within a reasonable period of time, abstract them accurately, and be capable of pulling ad hoc queries from the registry as needed are critical to the success of a high-performing performance improvement program.

© The Author(s), under exclusive license to Springer Nature Switzerland AG 2021   35
J. S. Young, *Trauma Center Performance Improvement*,
https://doi.org/10.1007/978-3-030-71048-4_6

Registry Leadership

The trauma registrar is a key position in a trauma center. This may be a nurse but often is not somebody with a nursing degree. The American College of Surgeons requires a certain amount of training for the registrar and quality control processes. The registrar will often report directly to the trauma program manager and will often have several direct reports. In some programs, the direct reports function merely as data abstractor's, while in other programs, there may be several registrars of fairly equal capabilities that can abstract, query, and help construct questions and answers for the PI program.

Routine Activities

The registrar is in charge of ensuring that the registry is accurate and up to date. The American College of Surgeons requires that the registry be current within 180 days of the current date. This is important because the registry is well, and Dave is unable to do up-to-date performance improvement activities. There are many training materials available for people interested in the nuts and bolts of the registry function. The registrar's basic activities are to look at the admit list from the previous day, identify injured patients, and begin the abstraction by recording demographic information from those patients' charts and information from the resuscitation and initial treatment. In some registries, the registrars go back daily to add data to the registry record. In others, they wait until the patient is discharged to do a final abstraction.

Periodically the registrar and the program manager will to quality control and pick random registry records and compare them to the data in the patient's medical record. There are also requirements for quality control for the American College of Surgeons Trauma Quality Improvement Project (TQIP).

The program may or may not review registry entries on a daily basis. I have inspected one or two programs where the trauma program manager reviewed every day's registry entries and did up-to-date performance improvement work on the patients while they were currently in the hospital. While this is the most up-to-date way, looking at patient care is also very demanding. In most centers, especially busy and mature centers, the trauma program has a weekly meeting usually with the program manager or the trauma PI coordinator, the registrar, and the physician responsible for PI to look at the patient that have come in in the previous week to see if any cases demand immediate analysis. In addition, as I said in previous chapters, this meeting is used to keep track of ongoing PI activities, update projects, and assign the task as they become available.

In the multidisciplinary performance improvement meeting that should be conducted monthly, it is extremely wise for the registry to generate a report that provides attendees with the basic information about admissions in the past month, the past quarter, and the current fiscal year. In addition, it should provide information on those subjects important to the program. These include how many helicopter transfers there were, how he transfers from specific hospitals, how many patients with injury severity scores above 25, and how many patients with the Glasgow coma score of 8 or less. It is useful to review these reports at the end of the MDPI meeting so that the entire group can look at the current data, and assess whether referrals are increasing or decreasing from certain areas,whether your unadjusted survival in different types of patients is changing, and, if you are a member of the national trauma databank or the trauma quality improvement project, update this presentation with the quarterly results from your benchmarking report.

Special Activities

Special activities include ad hoc queries that focus on subjects that are important to the program. These special projects can include audits of efficiency (e.g., time spent in ED), audits of previous PI events used for loop closure, and monitoring of the trauma program's basic performance. Your trauma registrar and the registry must be efficient at creating reports on the fly. If asking for something as simple as a list of severely injured patients who were admitted in July takes 3 weeks to receive, then you will not be able to make sophisticated improvement since you will likely forget that you even ask about the queries 3 weeks later.

Here are some examples of special queries and filters that the trauma registry can provide to the trauma program:

- Outcome of severely head-injured patients
- Time to femur fracture fixation
- Time to open tibia washout
- Time to antibiotics for open fractures
- Emergency department dwell time for highest-level activations
- Emergency department dwell time for lowest-level activations
- Percentage of time that a certain attending is present for the highest-level activation within 15 minutes
- Percentage of time that the trauma attendings present within 15 minutes for all highest-level activations
- Percentage of time the second-level activations are seen within 12 hours

Obviously, the list of possible registry queries is endless, and a program that has an extremely capable registry and registrar that can answer even a complex question quickly and accurately is a tremendous asset. I believe that every program should have an ad hoc query every month either based on opportunities for improvement or based on perceived inefficiencies in patient care. To do these queries, it is important to have excellent data integrity and very few missing fields in the registry reference. This is why a capable trauma registrar is so important and why a quality control program for the registry is essential.

Research Versus PI

There is often a fine line between registry performance improvement activities and research. In most US hospitals, their institutional review boards will allow research type activities under the umbrella of performance improvement. In these cases, should the results lead to the desire for publication, then a waiver of consent application should be made to the institutional review board. For those activities that start out as research questions where the goal from the beginning is to publish the results, you should contact the Official Review Board prior to beginning to look at data and determine whether consent is necessary or whether it can be waived. Remember, almost all research protocols have a defined time limit and usually need to be reviewed and extended on a yearly basis. Should the research not pan out, or the research question is no longer being investigated, you should shut down your research protocol.

In addition, many physicians, nurses, or other clinicians of the trauma center may want questions answered from the registry. The program should do everything they can to encourage this activity as it shows deep interest in the care of trauma patients and often curiosity as to the performance of these groups of clinicians. All requests such as this should be reviewed by the trauma program manager or the trauma medical director for approval for data retrieval. If necessary, trauma program personnel may need to request that the personnel that are asking for information go through the institutional review board to obtain permission before extracting the data from the registry. I believe that it shows an extremely lively trauma center with interested parties looking to improve themselves when you find that you are frequently being asked to provide quantitative data on injured patient care for your hospital.

In summary, the trauma registry is a critical and required part of every trauma program in any level trauma center. The registrar should be given sufficient time to carry out registry activities and should have sufficient personnel to be able to abstract charts; it is as close to real time as possible. The registrar should develop systems by which medical records are examined on a regular basis to determine if new data has appeared, and there should be rigorous quality control programs in place to ensure data integrity and that every field that can be filled in is filled in. Every trauma center should try to obtain benchmarking of the results. The trauma quality improvement program of the American College of Surgeons is probably the most respected benchmarking program available. There are others available, but you need to make certain that they are benchmarking against a large enough dataset to provide accurate risk adjustment. I would encourage every trauma center that wishes to determine whether they are providing optimal care to obtain benchmarking, and I would recommend the trauma quality improvement program since it is the most widely used in the United States.

There are several excellent resources and training courses in registry operations. Here are a few:

- Online trauma registry course provided by the American Trauma Society (https://www.amtrauma.org/page/TRC).
- The Trauma Registrar Mentoring Program by Pomphrey Consulting (https://www.pomphreyconsulting.com/traumaregistrar.html).
- The Trauma Registrar Advanced Prep Course by Pomphrey Consulting (https://www.pomphreyconsulting.com/store/p44/Trauma_Advanced_Registrar_Prep_%28TARP%29.html).

And many states publish trauma registry resources, for example:

- Colorado (https://www.colorado.gov/pacific/cdphe/trauma-registry-manual),
- Florida (http://www.floridahealth.gov/licensing-and-regulation/trauma-system/trauma-registry/_documents/Trauma-reg-manual-2016.pdf)
- and Kansas, among others (http://www.kstrauma.org/download/TraumaRegistrarGuide.pdf).

Chapter 7
Event Identification

There are many aspects of the chapter discussed previously, including identifying mortalities and using your registry to enhance your PI program. We discuss some additional specifics here that, for the most part, involve integration with your hospital safety program.

Safety Reporting (Hospital and Trauma Program)

All hospitals are required to have a safety reporting system. This usually entails an icon on each computer where any staff member can enter an event for further analysis and investigation. There are many products available for this, but they can allow the staff member to report anonymously. Still, an anonymous report cannot lead to an interview regarding the events and often is suboptimal.

The reports usually include technical and demographic information about where the event occurred, who the patient was, who the physicians or staff were, the circumstances of the event, and then what immediate discussion or corrective actions were taken to lessen the effect of the problem. These reports span a wide range of issues from incorrect meal trays all the way to failure to escalate and death. All hospitals have some sort of "quality" department that, in addition to looking at metrics and meeting all regulatory criteria, reviews these reports, and decides on further action follow-up for corrective action.

Most trauma programs do not have a specified computer application for reporting safety events. The most common method is direct communication with a member of the trauma program staff, escalating an issue through a specialty liaison, a manager of the clinical unit, manager of the support service, or email communications. In general, the hospital will receive a much larger amount of safety reports than the trauma program due to the hospital's larger size and the greater potential for issues.

One problem often identified during site visits is a lack of integration between the trauma program and the hospital quality program. In most cases, the trauma program will have a more advanced performance improvement process than the hospital, but there are hospitals that are fairly advanced in this area and will rival their trauma programs' efficiency and effectiveness. It is important that information flow both ways regarding safety issues for a variety of reasons. A safety issue may have impacted a trauma patient but could just as easily have affected a cardiology patient, and by having the information siloed within the trauma program, the corrective action cannot be generalized to other patient populations. Alternatively, hospital quality programs will usually have far more resources than the trauma PI program and can attack larger problems that span multiple areas of the hospital. The trauma program can usually contribute to these efforts significantly.

Most hospitals will have a method of routing reported issues that involve injured patients directly to the trauma PI program. There should also be a method for the trauma program to route issues that are beyond their scope to the hospital quality personnel for corrective action. This can get very confusing in the area of mortality. In most academic centers, the mortality may be assessed by the hospital quality program, the trauma program, and the individual medical/surgical specialty through morbidity and mortality conferences. It can often be very difficult to spread key findings in any of these three investigations. What occurs in our program is our trauma PI coordinator attends morbidity and mortality conferences when the trauma patient is being discussed so that he or she can bring this information back to the trauma investigation. The trauma program PI staff should always be included in root cause analyses or other interventions and data gathering events that the hospital quality program may execute. It is often a red flag to reviewers to see that critical issues that the trauma program identifies may affect other patients are not communicated to the hospital and vice versa. In your PI records, you should have communications with a hospital documented and included in the individual PI record. If the case is discussed at a hospital program meeting, if possible, the section of the minutes pertaining to this case should be included in the trauma PI records.

Sentinel Events

A sentinel event is a Patient Safety Event that reaches a patient and results in any of the following: death, permanent harm, or severe temporary harm and requires intervention. (https://www.jointcommission.org/resources/patient-safety-topics/sentinel-event/sentinel-event-policy-and-procedures/). Severe temporary harm or intervention required to sustain life can often be very difficult to identify as these are often referred to as "near misses." Often near misses may result from poor judgment, and the practitioners or staff may not be enthusiastic about reporting these issues if the patient recovered. This is why a "no blame" performance improvement environment is critical to improving care. Punishment is usually only reserved when staff is repeatedly informed of a requirement, acknowledges understanding of the rule, and continually violates this requirement. The staff that are carrying out their normal duties which may make an error in judgment, and unconscious medical error (dosing and medication errors, or misidentification of patients) must be encouraged to report these events by explaining that it is part of their ethos to ensure that a preventable error does not occur in another patient's care if it is avoidable.

Collection of Events

PI programs can cause themselves many problems by collecting more or fewer events than are necessary to improve the care delivered to the patient. I have inspected facilities where ~75% of their PI cases/issues involve events that (1) do not directly impact care, or (2) that involve issues that are better handled by human resources or another related department. Bad behavior in the trauma bay certainly needs to be addressed, but it is probably more important that those issues go through hospital human resources or physician staff office resources. Also, problems along these lines are difficult to solve (short of firing the person) since there is no real way for the trauma program to "audit" behavior, so behavior and interpersonal issues are better handled by other departments.

It is also very difficult to find and examine "near misses" unless they are directly reported to the hospital or trauma program. "Near misses" can provide more substrate for effective PI than even mortality, so it is important to find these events. Naturally, "near misses" may entail medical decision-making mistakes or errors of commission and omission. Unless observed by someone willing to report these events, it is somewhat unlikely that a clinician will report an issue that did not hurt the patient.

In no other area is it more important to have a "no blame" environment. No rational staff member will report an issue that no one else observed, did not harm the patient, and will lead to their firing. So a program must "advertise" to gather these events. Providing anonymous reporting is useful (however, it is often suboptimal to investigate an issue without speaking directly to the reporting staff member), or rewarding staff members for reporting "near misses" can encourage reporting. Many hospitals will provide gifts, money, or other incentives to those staff members that come forward to report dangerous problems. Of course, if the "near miss" was caused by a staff member's clear negligence, it should not be rewarded.

Initial Discussion

In some programs, the TMD is involved in every PI event, but that is impossible for busy programs. Usually, the PI coordinator and/or TPM will read about the event in whatever form it comes into the program (quality reporting software, email, conversation, etc.) and should try to contact the person reporting the event to gather the information that may degrade with time. This can be an obvious problem in an anonymously reported event (we will go into anonymous reporting further in the discussion of personal issues).

Once the event is reviewed and initial information gathered, the event should be triaged (see next chapter). Triage may direct the process to an immediate discussion with the TMD, insertion into the death review process, aggregation into a file of similar events with a coordinated PI process, etc.

Some events (medication errors, catheter-associated urinary tract infection (CAUTI), central line infections (CLABSI), falls, etc.) will require hospital quality program integration and investigation, and the program should inform the hospital department of the event to ensure they were able to pick it up. Deaths should have their own process with thorough and immediate registry file completion, review of the patient record, gathering of information on final events leading to demise, discussion with TPM (for cases that can be easily triaged to anticipated without (OFI), i.e., a gunshot wound to head presenting with GCS 3 and no patient-initiated breaths that go on to organ donation) with rapid confirmation of the categorization by the TMD, or elevation to a weekly PI or trauma service discussion with secondary triage from those meetings.

Chapter 8
Levels of Review

Examples

There are several rubrics to triage PI issues, but the method we use categorizes events by these:

- Does the issue have the potential to cause serious harm?
- Does the issue have the potential to affect a large number of patients?

Those issues that meet both criteria require "emergent" intervention, often consisting of ad hoc meetings, rapid improvement events, and the involvement of those executives who could rapidly implement corrective actions. The next triage group would be those who meet one of the criteria. The next group would be little harm, but that can affect many patients.

Here are some examples and suggested triage:

- An OR staff member hooked an oxygen line to a CO_2 outlet in an OR room. A trauma patient underwent surgery and rapidly became hypoxic. The patient was taken off the ventilator and was bag masked using a separate oxygen tank. The saturations immediately came up, but when the patient was put back on the ventilator, the hypoxia recurred. The anesthesiologist felt this could be an anesthesia machine problem and ventilated off an auxiliary tank. The operation went fine, but afterward, the mistake was found.

  - This is a critical error that could have caused serious harm to the patient and could harm others. This is the highest-level event. Anesthesia, clinical engineering, and hospital administration were called to an immediate meeting. All walked down to the OR and looked at the hookups. Though the CO_2 outlet was clearly marked in yellow and the oxygen in green, the connector would fit on either outlet. This was felt to be unacceptable. Several other institutions were immediately contacted, and there is an equipment solution where an

J. S. Young, *Trauma Center Performance Improvement*,
https://doi.org/10.1007/978-3-030-71048-4_8

adaptor can be placed on the outlet and hose such that it can only be hooked to the CO2 outlet and not the oxygen outlet. It would take a week to obtain the equipment and install it; thus, an immediate safety solution was needed. An emergency meeting was held for all OR staff the following morning at 6 AM, where the event was discussed and the solution outlined. This warned all staff. Also, since CO2 outlets were only in five operating rooms, a cover was placed over each of these outlets with a large, brightly colored warning. The equipment was installed the following week, and there were no further similar events.

- A massive transfusion protocol is initiated for two patients with gunshot wounds in the ED within 5 minutes of each other. Both patients are anonymous and have unknown patient designations (in our facility, they are assigned a letter, gender, and country, for instance, B-Male, England). The blood coolers arrive simultaneously, and a unit was removed from each cooler. One patient was severely hypotensive and moving to OR, and blood was hung as he left without checking. When checking the blood for the second patient, it was realized that the coolers were switched (even though the same type of blood is in each cooler, the blood is assigned to an MRN, so if there is a reaction, the blood administered can be tracked and of course for other reasons). The OR was called, and the coolers were switched back, and the blood bank was informed.

  - This was not triaged as high as the previous case, but it was jumped on within 24 hours, and the corrective action plan was created within 7 days, and all actions were complete within 30 days. This is an example of a situation where no harm came to the patient, but significant harm could come to the next patient if they were given type and crossed blood from another patient. The investigation revealed inconsistent practices when checking massive transfusion protocol blood and even crossmatched blood in a hyper-urgent situation. So the entire blood checking process was dissected with the frontline ICU, ED, and OR personnel. It was found that for MTP, blood labels could be more clearly placed on the blood indicating the patient and that the blood bank would also put a taped note on the outside of each cooler indicating which patient that cooler was intended for. It was also stressed that blood must be checked in all situations, and a unit of blood should never just be grabbed out of a cooler and transfused without checking some items in any situation since a mistake could be as fatal as the patient's primary problem. Education and simulation were carried out with ED, ICU, and anesthesia personnel, and further refinements were made with feedback.

- An 87-year-old patient suffers a ground-level fall. The patient suffers a femur fracture, pelvic fracture, and multiple rib fractures, as well as a T5 compression fracture. The patient suffers a catheter associated urinary tract infection (CAUTI) during their 10-day stay and a hospital-acquired pressure ulcer (HAPU).

– This is a good example of a case where the trauma program and the hospital quality program can integrate activities. All US hospitals track and investigate CAUTI and HAPU. It is possible that the trauma program may not catch these complications, and the hospital program would not communicate it in a timely manner. Therefore, it is important that the PI leads for the trauma program and the registrar establish data and personal relationships with their hospital counterparts. In this case, there are likely already established guidelines for urinary catheter use and the prevention of pressure ulcers. The nursing units will usually carry out an initial investigation to look for problems mobilizing the patient and whether a urinary catheter was in place longer than it needed to be or if there was a break in insertion and/or maintenance technique. The trauma program should track these hospital events and include them in the patient's PI record as well as on its dashboard. TQIP also tracks these events, and this allows the program to compare its event rate to other hospitals in the program. So, in this case, the program and hospital would work together to investigate, analyze, and determine and implement corrective action. One problem that often appears on-site visits is that an issue is sent to the hospital quality program, and information is never circled back. This is a problem for the trauma program because this will appear to the site visitors as an open loop or an example that the PI program is delegating PI activities to the hospital program to avoid dealing with them. Either way, it is vital that the trauma program complete loop closure, even if it means tracking down the hospital investigation and forcing them to share their findings so they can be included in the trauma program loop closure documentation.

From these cases, you can learn that events where there is harm and which have a high chance of recurrence must be addressed immediately. Events involving medical decision-making in complex patients have a longer timeline, and events that reflect system conditions requiring extensive collaboration for forming an action plan and the involvement of multiple services in the corrective action plan will require more time.

Deaths

There is some variability in the levels of review of deaths. What is consistent is that all deaths must be reviewed, but some programs will allow the TPM to completely evaluate expected mortality with no OFI (i.e., prehospital traumatic arrest with short-term return of vital signs and a fatal gunshot wound to the brain) have the TMD sign off on review, and present in tabular form at the trauma center multidisciplinary PI meeting (MDPI). Other centers have a set process of levels of review of deaths and follow this for all cases. For immature centers, all deaths should be reviewed in the same manner: event discovery, initial chart abstraction, and performance improvement personnel review along with gathering frangible information from frontline staff, if a clinical issue review by another trauma faculty not involved in the case (can be optional in some centers as long as you do not have final review authority on your own cases). The process is a formal presentation to the TPM and physician PI lead, assessment for OFI and corrective actions, the initial recommendation for preventability, and formal presentation at peer review and MDPI.

Adverse Events

The FDA defines an adverse event as any undesirable experience associated with the use of a medical product in a patient. In general, hospitals widen this definition to include any undesirable experience in the hospital, but routine patient complaints that do not involve deficits in care are usually handled by another pathway (https://www.fda.gov/safety/reporting-serious-problems-fda/what-serious-adverse-event).

Adverse event investigation can be very difficult in many centers. Assume that there is not a member of the trauma program staff integrated with daily rounds. In that case, it can be hard to identify adverse events that fall beyond the common ones monitored by most hospitals (falls with injury, CAUTI, CLABSI, HAPU, etc.). In addition, near misses can be very difficult to identify, especially during off-hours. A hospital must have an extremely robust quality reporting system with totally blameless investigations in order to prompt staff to report near misses.

There are more examples of adverse events than can be listed here, but in the trauma world, they include the following:

• Medication errors
• Equipment malfunctions
• Delays in diagnosis
• Errors of omission and commission
• Ventilator-associated pneumonia
• Osteomyelitis
• Wound infection

Adverse events usually are signals of system issues (a piece of equipment is not being used properly, a problem with accurate medication reconciliation, low respiratory therapy staffing in the ICU, etc.). Every admission likely has some untoward event (e.g., ordering a CT for within 4 hours and it not being done for 8 hours), but many do not cause patient harm. A trauma program can tie itself in knots pursuing every care defect since perfect medical care is a fantasy. What is not fantasy is being very diligent in examining the care you are delivering and continually improving it. Some site reviewers will look at every adverse event as an indication of overall poor care; however, this is not the way this should be evaluated. If a critical error happens over and over and is either not discovered, analyzed, or corrected, this can definitely indicate a problem with overall care delivery. However, single adverse events happen in even the strongest and safest care systems. They merely need to be discovered, analyzed, and corrected. It is not poor PI to determine that an adverse event resulted from such an unusual confluence of circumstances that corrective action is not needed; however, this decision should be thoroughly documented in the PI records, and there should be evidence that the underlying components of care are solid.

Adverse events should undergo the same PDSA process as a PI issue. The ACS asks for charts that reflect adverse events in the ICU, however; however, multiple adverse events that happen anywhere in the continuum of care can be aggregated into a completed PI project that should be presented to site reviewers. We discuss adverse events that result from poor decision-making or clinician performance later in this chapter.

System Issues

System issues may represent critical problems within a trauma center. The ACS requires a separate system-based agenda and meeting, though many programs integrate system discussion and analysis into their regularly scheduled PI meeting, the only difference is that the system portion of the meeting will require additional representation from EMS, laboratory, blood bank, etc.

System issues usually require a multidisciplinary approach to correction. By definition, the word "system" indicates that the problem crosses multiple services and departments. System issues also include EMS as well as post-acute care facilities. System issues can also be difficult correct in that it requires the cooperation of multiple departments and hospital services. The maxim "Perfect is the greatest enemy of good" should be applied to these issues. It may not be feasible to spend the time and effort to correct the problem that has been vexing the hospital for decades but rather spend a focused effort on creating a good solution that improves trauma patients' care.

A system issue example that we have faced for many years is a notification by EMS in a timely manner, more specifically, aeromedical services. In our system, all EMS communications go through MEDCOM, which is a service within the hospital staffed by paramedics that both take incoming EMS communications and dispatche helicopter services as needed. These paramedics monitor our area of the state and are usually aware of the helicopters being dispatched to a scene. For anyone who has done EMS, they know that it can often be difficult for the crew caring for the patient to take the time to give a detailed report to the hospital before arrival. However, in trauma systems, some accurate data is needed to assign activation levels and gather necessary personnel and equipment properly. A maxim I like to use is "if you're only ready when you're needed, then you're not ready," meaning that if the trauma team arrives coincident with the appearance of the patient and the trauma bay, then problems usually ensue.

We have found through cause analysis of emergency department errors that the most common cause identified is late notification and activating a high-level alert only after the patient arrives in the emergency department. When that happens, there is usually a disjointed primary and secondary survey in that the emergency medicine physicians begin the survey or may begin therapy as it is proper for them to do. Then the trauma team shows up in the middle of this and has to reorient themselves to the condition of the patient and often repeat the primary and secondary survey and may initiate therapy that could be different from what the emergency medicine physician started. Regardless it invariably creates confusion, poor information flow, and inefficient resuscitation.

When we analyzed these cases, we found that when the helicopter was dispatched to a scene, we often received a report within 5 minutes of arrival. This did not provide adequate time to assemble the trauma team and to put out an alert page. On further analysis, we found that often the helicopters in the air for 20 to 25 minutes prior to giving the report. Thus, we undertook a lengthy and ongoing PI project where we brought in representatives of all the helicopter services as well as chief officers from local EMS agencies to describe to them the problem we are facing and ask for solutions. Some solutions that were implemented were a voice-activated headset for the paramedic with the patient so that they did not need to leave the patient to pick up a radio microphone and can merely click a button to talk to the hospital; we also encourage cellular phone communication since this was direct and go on to a recorded line for further qualitative analysis. We audited for an entire year "trauma alert now" activations, which are set off when the patient's arrival is expected within 10 minutes. We were able to demonstrate that the incidence of these "trauma alert now" activations decreased and when they did occur were appropriate and that the patient was local and there was not more than 10 minutes warning available.

Another example is the way that our activation system works. In our facility, MEDCOM receives the communication but could not activate an alert unless approved by the emergency medicine physician. For many years, it was difficult and time-consuming to page the emergency medicine attending. This resulted in delays and activation that were truly unnecessary. The patient clearly met the criteria for activation in front of the MEDCOM operator when they took the call. We tried several technological solutions, including a direct connection phone and radios, but occasional problems still appeared. After lengthy conversations with emergency medicine, it was decided that if the communication received by the paramedics clearly indicated the highest-level activation by the criteria, they could activate the alert and notify the emergency medicine attending afterward. For a second-level activation "beta," they were still required to contact emergency medicine attending. But if after 3 minutes, they could not make contact, they could activate the alert based on the criteria. We still continue to monitor this and have improved performance over time.

Another example of a complex system issue is ED dwell times. I have said many lectures that when someone mentions the amount of time their highest-level activation,patients spend in the emergency department, and people in the audience go, "that's crazy our patients don't spend that much time in the ED," I tell them do not say that until you have actually seen your data. In my podcasts on clinicalbraintraining.com, I described "inertia" in the care of the trauma patient. This involves wasting small but significant increments of time before a patient is transferred to the ICU that accumulates, sometimes in excess of 2 hours.

To tackle this problem requires a truly multidisciplinary approach. Delays in the ED may be due to bed availability, OR availability, radiology throughput issues, inefficiency in deciding on the proper workup, or repeating tests due to suboptimal decisions made during the initial evaluation. I will describe all of the measures we took to try to improve this (and we still struggle with this issue to this day), but solutions included always having an "alpha" bed available in the surgical intensive care unit such that a critical patient could come up from the emergency department immediately. We also implemented a variety of alerts that notify critical personnel such as the nursing supervisor, the ICU manager, the OR manager, and relevant specialties for certain conditions that require coordination of multiple services such as an operative head injury.

System issues that are analyzed effectively and where prudent corrective actions are put in place that demonstrate improvement are extremely impressive to site visit teams. They indicate that the trauma program can cross departmental and service lines to correct problems. It is less impressive to the team when significant system issues are not corrected due to turf battles and poor interactions between critical personnel.

Personal Issues

I want to spend some time here talking about personal issues and involve the trauma PI program. Regarding physician behavior, I believe that the systems that are already in place in every hospital, which include the medical staff office, and the chief medical officer, should be used for issues where a physician is acting inappropriately toward patients or toward other personnel. The only role of the trauma PI program would be those attendings within the trauma surgery division to require redirection and corrective action. However, it is likely even in these physicians that complaints about behavior will need to go through the hospital process.

I had evaluated trauma programs where clearly 40% of the PI issues in their PI log represented people being mean to each other, yelling when things were not available, or yelling when there were delays in care. Even though this is certainly suboptimal for the care of the patient that so many issues arose with clinicians, it more likely reflects problems with the trauma system itself. Whenever you see that a physician is constantly being angered by what goes on resuscitation day, it could be a personal issue, but it also could be a serious defect in the way the resuscitations are conducted and whether necessary equipment and consultants are readily available. When the program sees multiple personnel issues in a service area or between departments, they need to not reflexively attribute this to bad personalities (even though this may be the root cause) but need to examine the process of providing care and query the people involved to get to the cause of the issue. We have found in our experience that often the poor personal interaction as a result of a clinician facing the same dumb issue over and over and despite trying to work toward solutions finding it is still not fixed. Nothing is quite as worrisome to a site visit team evaluating the PI program than significant issues that are brought up multiple times that show no progress toward resolution. Assume that you have issues such as this within your system that is resistant to correction due to political or other considerations within your facility. You need to be frank with the site visitors about what is going on. If these are central to good patient care, then your hospital should reevaluate whether it should even be a trauma center since the ability to solve problems across departments and service areas is integral to providing optimal care for the injured patient.

Chapter 9
Documentation of PI Process and Meeting Minutes

What Is the Minimum Documentation?

A horrible outcome of a site visit would be one where you have an effective, organized, and mature PI program but receive a criterion deficiency because your minutes and records are poor. Creating minutes is time-consuming and often unrewarded because, as we all know, when minutes are approved at subsequent meetings, they are rarely read. However, minutes are critical in demonstrating that you have effective PI meetings, that you push event analysis and correction forward, and that you close loops. It can also be helpful with vexing problems that you cannot solve by demonstrating to the reviewers how hard you are trying to improve, and it also demonstrates to them who is being an obstacle to change.

Most meetings are recorded and transcribed in some fashion. A word-by-word retelling of the meeting is not necessary. You should include the agenda, attendance, specific issues discussed, the heart of the discussion, the next steps, and who is assigned to move this forward. Adding a due date for a deliverable is also an excellent component of the minutes. Examples will be provided later in this chapter.

There are some states where peer review documents are discoverable, thus virtually ensuring that a frank retelling of the meeting will not exist. However, centers in these states still need to demonstrate to the site visit team the work they are doing and cannot simply say, "we don't create minutes because they are discoverable." Centers have come up with many solutions. First, you should consult with your hospital attorneys to confirm exactly what is discoverable and in what setting. Even in states with broad access, there can still be protection for sensitive documents. Next, you need to stand back and analyze exactly what parts of the PI records are critical to demonstrate progress. Is the patient's name, age, and day of admission really necessary? They are not; patients can be anonymized either with a false name, a number, or some other method. Ages can be generalized (60–65-year-old etc.). But as you can see, this can become very complicated.

J. S. Young, *Trauma Center Performance Improvement*,
https://doi.org/10.1007/978-3-030-71048-4_9

A solution that may satisfy reviewers is to demonstrate what cases were reviewed (which should not be an issue if discovered) and then take the OFIs that are found and separate these from the cases that generated them. For instance, if a specific death revealed a problem with communication for the massive transfusion protocol at your institution, take that OFI and perform a PI project on that issue alone. The OFIs can even be coded, so they cannot be traced back to individual cases.

As you can see, this is somewhat burdensome, but trauma surgeons did not write these laws, and when you view this from the vantage of the ACS COT, we cannot simply give centers in these states a pass when they cannot demonstrate the effectiveness of their PI program. Reviewers will usually be lenient with regard to tracing issues back to specific cases but still will need to see PDSA cycles being applied.

Thus minimum documentation is as follows:

1. Agenda, date, and time
2. Attendance
3. Concise writeup of the discussion (but try your best to preserve the key elements of the discussion, for instance, if a specific provider's actions are in question, the discussion of those actions and especially the comments of the treating clinician are critical to demonstrate the program is willing to hold difficult conversations on sensitive issues)
4. Outcomes of discussion

   (a) Closure
   (b) Auditing
   (c) Education
   (d) Protocol development
   (e) Specific communication to providers
   (f) Escalation to hospital program

5. Responsible person
6. Due date for deliverable or update

As you can see, this is another reason why trivial issues should not be brought to the mandatory PI meeting. You need to spend your time on OFIs that may have led to patient harm and system issues that are consistently causing suboptimal care.

Templates

Coordination Systems

Although trauma programs for many years worked with just the TMD and TPM coordinating the PI program, even modest-sized programs will find it very difficult to have an organized PI process without additional personnel. Often, the surgeon who is being groomed to eventually succeed the TMD will be given the role of PI medical director (or some other similar title). This allows this surgeon to begin to understand the PI process and to learn how to interact with other specialties and units concerning PI issues. Most often, a nurse is appointed PI coordinator (or a similar title). This person coordinates all PI activities, performs investigations, creates PI records, and organizes the monthly PI meeting. Of course, the TPM assists with these activities, but many programs work with a PI coordinator controlling all PI activities. It is important for either of these personnel to be properly trained through a TOPIC course or through an extended apprenticeship observing the TPM and TMD. In the latest revisions of the ACS optimal resources document, a 0.5 FTE dedicated to PI will be required in smaller programs, and a full FTE will be required in busier centers.

Whoever is the lead for PI must develop a system to keep track of issues, find obstructions to loop closure (and work to overcome them), and document progress and loop closure in an easy-to-find and timely manner.

They will also be responsible for identifying cases for PI analysis and action and getting them on the agenda in as short a time as possible. One problem many programs have is getting way behind in PI cases. I have done site visits when unanticipated deaths from 12 months prior are still not closed, and this does not look good. At our program, in addition to our multidisciplinary PI meeting, we have two other weekly meetings: first is a PI meeting every Tuesday afternoon with the TPM, PI coordinator, Associate TMD for PI, administrative assistant, and a representative from the registry. At the conference, we review all highest-level activations from the week, major complications, deaths, and whatever system issues we are working on (MCI preparation, communications, laboratory issues, etc.) since this is an extremely effective method for disseminating information.

Situational Awareness of Open Issues

It is very easy for cases to fall behind. For certain issues, such as unanticipated deaths with OFI, it is very important to stay on track. Some of these cases have OFIs that can affect future patients' outcomes, so they must be addressed in a timely manner. Remember that a program must triage its work. The highest level should be urgent safety issues that are harming patients; right below that would be unanticipated deaths, then anticipated deaths with OFI, then deaths without OFI, then the rest. Sometimes a lower-level issue must be moved up because you are coordinating with hospital PI or for some other reason. But remember that cases that indicate patient harm are your highest priority.

Another strategy that we use is an aggregation of similar OFIs into a PI project. For instance, if you have an issue with administering splenic immunizations in splenectomy patients prior to discharge, instead of writing and collating 10 cases where this issue occurred, it is appropriate to write under the OFI in each chart "see splenic vaccine PI project" and then create a folder for this specific aggregated OFI. You can put the loop closure for the project in the project folder to demonstrate loop closure.

Review of Opportunities for Improvement

It is very easy for a program to lose track of opportunities for improvement and have them fester for months or years. This is especially true of OFIs that require crucial conversations or aware there has been significant resistance to change. The program must be aware that the site visit team will be looking for these types of issues and will be assessing how you handle them. It is not expected that the program is able to solve every problem because no trauma center can; however, it is expected that you do not simply ignore complex problems and cross them off your list.

As I said previously, it is important for the program to keep a running tab of opportunities for improvement that includes the date that the EOF I was found, the initial discussion, the responsible party for closing EOF I, a reasonable date of closure, follow-up, and loop closure documents. As I said in the previous section aggregating similar OFIs into projects can really simplify this problem. Each program handles this differently. In some programs, the trauma program managers are able to keep all of these issues in his or her head, but this is obviously not a good solution for the majority of programs. The most common method that I have seen is a log presented at the beginning of the multidisciplinary peer review meeting (or at the end) where the group looks at those opportunities that are still open and refuse the loop closure of those that seem to be able to be closed. It can be somewhat unwieldy for a busy program to go through all of these issues at their MDPI meeting since any busy program will have 10 or 15 issues in various stages of correction. It is important at the large meeting to go over those opportunities that have been stubborn to correct, require buy-in from multiple departments or areas, or where new protocol guidelines are put in place to close the loop. An example in our program has been our massive transfusion protocol. This protocol is in constant evolution, and in the case section, I will go over some of the paths that we have taken, but it is quite common for the blood bank to play a major role in our large PI meetings in that the function of the massive transfusion protocol is vital to saving lives and is quite complex and resource-intensive, and the program should be looking for ways to maximize effect while minimizing resources.

It is very important to be able to clearly demonstrate to the site visit team how you identified an issue, how you analyzed it, how you investigated it, and then how you carried out loop closure. While the site visitors spent time going to the actual facts of the case, many of us will take these facts off of the PI documents and merely check the actual record. By going off the documents, we are able to identify what issues the program itself felt were important or were not important. This gives us a good insight into how the performance improvement program works at the trauma center. You should expect that no site visit team will take a single case and try to hang you with in it. Every trauma center has cases that they are not proud of and where they face political issues that they cannot overcome. It is the response to these cases that is most important and which demonstrates the diligence of the trauma program in trying to improve care. Many examples of PI documents will be given in the case section.

Chapter 10
Loop Closure

What Does Loop Closure Mean?

Loop closure is the method where you take an opportunity for improvement and institute a corrective action plan and demonstrate that the corrective action plan is likely to prevent a recurrence of this problem. Loop closure can take many forms. Some opportunities can be closed by the trauma program manager, while some require month-long multispecialty, multiunit discussions, guideline drafts, and complex implementation strategies.

This will be the longest chapter in this handbook, and for a good reason. Performance improvement without loop closure is, for the most part, a wasted activity. Identifying problems and analyzing them but not putting in measures to fix them does not improve care. The most frequently cited deficiency during site visits is an absent or inconsistent loop closure.

The nature of the opportunity often determines the method of loop closure. Personal issues can often be solved by education and reprimand (which must be documented). Equipment and supply issues can be corrected through work with the relevant services and units to change equipment storage and availability and education. Ventilator-associated pneumonia, urinary tract infection, and other common complications can have their loop close by examining if aspects of the recommended practice were not done, why, and looking at the tools used and revising if necessary.

Can You Close All Loops?

The answer to this question is no. It is impossible to close all opportunities for improvement with solid loop closure. Now many programs may appear to be closing all are loops through the ubiquitous use of education and discussion for problems where those two methods of loop closure are not optimal. But in most programs, they will do their best to close as many lives as possible, close all loops that endanger the patient, and have reasonable explanations for other issues that do not get completely resolved. But as we all know, some issues cannot always be resolved. Certain physician issues need to be ameliorated through discussion of a clinician supervisor, education and the clinician, and monitoring of care. I have seen institutions where a certain clinician has enough political power in their institution that they cannot be removed from the trauma panel. Any experience trauma director knows that these situations do exist and the medical director may not always have it within their power to correct them. In these situations, it is important that the PI program thoroughly document the efforts that were put in. Through thorough documentation, the site visit team can bring this issue up to executive management, which may help the program close the loop. However, it is not a good idea to expect to use the site visit as a tool for addressing opportunities for improvement.

To reiterate, adverse events or opportunities for improvement that cause adverse outcomes or could apply to large numbers of patients must be addressed. It is unacceptable for a trauma center to leave in place a clinician or process that endangers patients. There are criterion deficiencies available to the American College of Surgeons site review team that can be used to indicate that the hospital has an insufficient dedication to trauma. This insufficient dedication is evidenced by the fact that despite pleading from the trauma program, executive management will not make an effort to correct the problem. This is a very serious deficiency, and if you have issues in this realm, you must do everything in your power to try to correct them and document these efforts.

Loop Closure Methods

Discussion

Discussion is commonly used as a method of loop closure. At the very least, the discussions need to be documented with the date and personnel in attendance. You also should document the content of the discussion as thoroughly as possible. Site visit teams will not look kindly on the discussion being used as a method of loop closure for a poorly designed process. Knowledge of performance improvement teaches us that badly designed processes cannot be overcome through sheer force of will. Thus discussing the defects in a badly designed process without trying to correct the process is bad PI. If the discussion takes place with the provider, whether it be a nurse, physician assistant, a surgeon, or any other clinician who has behaved badly or is consistently ignoring the care guidelines set forth by the trauma program, this should be thoroughly documented with the time, place, and should indicate that the clinician understood the content of the discussion and vowed to prevent recurrence.

Many cases are closed at morbidity and mortality conferences through discussion (in fact, this is obviously the most common form of closure in a surgery M&M conference). This is because physician judgment is very difficult to review retrospectively. Intraoperative misadventures often cannot be corrected through protocol development. What a surgeon decides to do with a certain injury can be controlled within the specialty, but that is often beyond what the trauma director can do unless it happens to be in the realm of general surgery or surgical critical care. The program should do its best to control variability through guideline development and evidence-based medicine with daily rounds in discussions of complex patients. If the practitioner is consistently performing outside except the parameters, it is incumbent upon the programs to remove the practitioner from the call panel or to demonstrate that corrective action has been effective.

Education

I cannot stress enough that education cannot be the solution to all opportunities for improvement. When you use education as a corrective action, you need to think to yourself: will this corrective action plan actually prevent this from happening in the future? Also, does education to a small group of providers ensure that anyone who may come in contact with the future patient will not repeat the mistake? Also, will education prevent an error in the middle of the night or when there is a high workload.

As I have said before, education will likely be the most common form of corrective action because it is simple to execute. However, you need to think long and hard before using education as corrective action for an opportunity for improvement that would cause moderate to severe patient harm and which could not reasonably be tied to a single provider. If the opportunity resulted from confusion, infrastructure problems, logistics, bed management, medication error, or procedural error, it is unlikely that an email or grand rounds are sufficient to ensure this will not recur.

When using education as a corrective action plan, it is imperative that the program provides the substance of the educational offering in their PI records, indicates when and where the education was provided, and has a record of who received the education. This is easier to do than it sounds. If grand rounds are given, you simply need to provide the slides for the grand rounds and the attendance list. An optimal educational offering would also include a posttest to indicate comprehension, but this is not absolutely necessary in all situations.

When the American College of Surgeons used the internal educational program as a continuing medical education substitute and as a tool for PI, many programs developed innovative solutions. My own program developed an online testing system where cases were presented, analyzed, lessons learned, and corrective actions were all presented, and posttest and responses were recorded. Other centers used pamphlets or emails with posttests. Some other centers used grand rounds and educational conferences with follow-up testing as well. But I have to say that since the IEP was removed as a CME substitute, many programs have moved away from sophisticated educational offerings, which is unfortunate because I thought they could be a very effective tool. However, there is nothing keeping you from using an internal educational program as a corrective action mechanism for opportunities for improvement.

The best educational offerings are those which instruct providers about evidence-based medicine concepts or newly developed protocols and guidelines. Moreover, remember that these discussions must be documented.

There are many possible examples of using education as a loop closure action. For example, if the patient is admitted without a CTA of the neck with multiple cervical spine fractures who goes on to develop a vascular event from an injury to the carotid artery, grand rounds refocused a set of slides developed using evidence-based guidelines for CTA of the neck can be developed. This can be presented in a grand round setting, but it would be better to have each clinician (surgeons and advanced practice practitioners and residents if applicable) receive the slides and have to do a posttest. In addition, for issues that are related to the workup of a trauma patient, emergency medicine should always be included. Also, for an offering such as this, you should show it to your radiology experts and ensure that they agree with the indications you are educating about. However, if you think on this more extensively, a guideline that is put in place where a CTA of the neck will be ordered if any of a number of injuries are identified in the cervical spine would be better loop closure. A communications process built into that new guideline where radiologists would directly contact a senior member of the trauma team if the cervical studies reveal a worrisome injury would possibly be even more effective. Also, if this error led to an adverse patient outcome, it would be beneficial for certain injuries to be audited for a period of time to ensure that no patients who should receive the CTA of the neck are falling through the cracks. Of course, you cannot do an extensive loop closure project on every issue, but those issues where an error can lead to a devastating patient outcome warrant the extra effort.

Personal Intervention

Misbehavior by clinicians (especially surgeons) is a fact of life. Even if you are lucky enough to have personnel that acts professionally in all situations, even the most friendly and teambuilding clinician can go off the rails in a high-pressure situation where multiple things are going wrong. In fact, sometimes, in those types of situations, it is necessary for the team leader to raise their voice and take control of the situation through whatever means they have at their disposal in order to redirect the team. But in the PI realm, we are referring to personnel specific cannot get along with others, or his behavior is disruptive to the team and potentially injurious to the patient. Every program and every hospital have guidelines for dealing with inappropriate behavior, and sometimes if the behavior is bad enough, it will be reported up to the hospital chain of command, and those protocols will be implemented. Sometimes it even leads to the dismissal of the physician or clinician. But for those instances where the trauma program gets involved, it will usually require the trauma medical director trauma program manager to interface with the supervisor of the clinician who was misbehaving. While there are instances where you can certainly go directly to the clinician and have a professional conversation about the need to act to benefit the patient (and that should often be your first step), a discussion with the supervisor is fairly routine. For nonphysicians, there is usually a tighter rein on bad behavior, and it is far less tolerated. However, for physicians, there can be problems. I have site visited centers where there are innumerable reports in the PI records of, for instance, a trauma surgeon disrupting the team in the emergency department. Also, in some instances, these surgeons are excellent clinicians, and the program is not excited about taking them off the call schedule. The trauma medical director needs to realize that if you can redirect this clinician through discussion, it will often positively affect their career path. For physicians who are constantly being reprimanded by their division chiefs, department chairs, or chief medical officer's tenure at your institution will usually be limited. Also, some of these physicians have difficulty finding jobs at other hospitals since it is routine to contact the clinical staff office of the previous hospital to see if there are any problems. Many programs exist to deal with physician behavior, and there is an excellent program at Vanderbilt University that you can obtain more information about. But these programs are usually residential offerings, are very expensive, and will take the physician out of commission for several weeks. As I said previously, being a trauma medical director in these types of situations can be the most uncomfortable part of the job. I work in an academic setting, so dealing with disruptive residences somewhat easier, but dealing with senior physicians on specialty services can be very frustrating. It is important for the trauma medical director to set the example of how one should conduct themselves during the trauma response patient, in the operating room, and during rounds. If the clinician's behavior rises to be reported to the PI program, then the same path of analysis, information gathering, and loop closure need to apply. Documentation of discussion in these types of situations is an adequate loop closure device, but as I said previously, trivial efforts will usually have trivial results. Recurring bad behavior will need to be escalated by the trauma program up to the clinical staff or staffing structure of the hospital.

On some site visits, I have seen PI programs where a large percentage of their opportunities for improvement involve personal interaction. First, this would indicate a hospital where most people would not work, but second, it shows that clinician behavior is out of control. It is hard to imagine that optimal patient care is being delivered when trauma resuscitations are screaming matches. In situations such as these may require the trauma program to get help to fix the problem. However, if everyone is angry at each other, the program should entertain the idea that the staff does not want to take care of trauma patients and that perhaps if it is possible, they should allow the patient to go somewhere else and give up on the idea of being a trauma center. This is a nuclear option, obviously, and a lot of effort should go into fixing this before you come to that conclusion, but I have seen instances where that was the conclusion, and it was best for everyone, including the patient. These types of interactions can also occur when a clinician from " a different background" (such as parts of the country where more direction forceful personal interactions are common). In these instances, it usually just takes time and peer pressure for that person to conform to their new surroundings.

Equipment Alterations

It is not uncommon for the trauma program to have to deal with faulty or unavailable equipment. This also includes instances where radiological studies were unavailable (indicating a shortage of X-ray equipment).

We had many issues with the availability of needed equipment in the resuscitation bay. Loop closure of these issues can be difficult because the trauma program does not usually have authority over the ED purchasing and storage. We came up with a unique solution for our center that has worked well for almost 10 years. A trauma cart was created by our trauma program manager Kathy Butler (Fig. 10.1) that contained all the necessary supplies for a trauma resuscitation.

As you can see the cart easy to move between rooms is stopped and walked by our central supply service, and all equipment is readily available. I will pretend it did not take a great deal of effort to implement the solution but it has worked extremely well. Another positive offshoot of portable trauma cart is the hospital response to multiple casualty incidents. We have 15 of these carts stored in our supply area in the basement of the hospital. In essence, rolling this car next to a hospital bed that has a monitor essentially makes that bed a trauma resuscitation bay. We have had multiple casualty incidents where these carts were rolled to various beds in our emergency department, greatly expanding our capacity for trauma resuscitation.

More commonly, equipment issues that arise to the performance improvement committee include lack of availability of things such as scalpels, appropriately sized chest tubes, sutures, and staplers. As stated above by creating a solution where recommended equipment were all stored in one place, they can be brought to the bedside, and we were able to close many of these loops with one project.

When equipment problems are reported up through the chain of command, it is important to determine whether this was a "one-off" situation which is not likely to occur, or this is a problem with stocking and availability. It is important at this point to engage the emergency department management and representatives from your central supply department to determine whether there is adequate stock of this piece of equipment in the emergency department, and if not how many are required and how often should their stock level be checked.

Fig. 10.1 Picture of current trauma cart

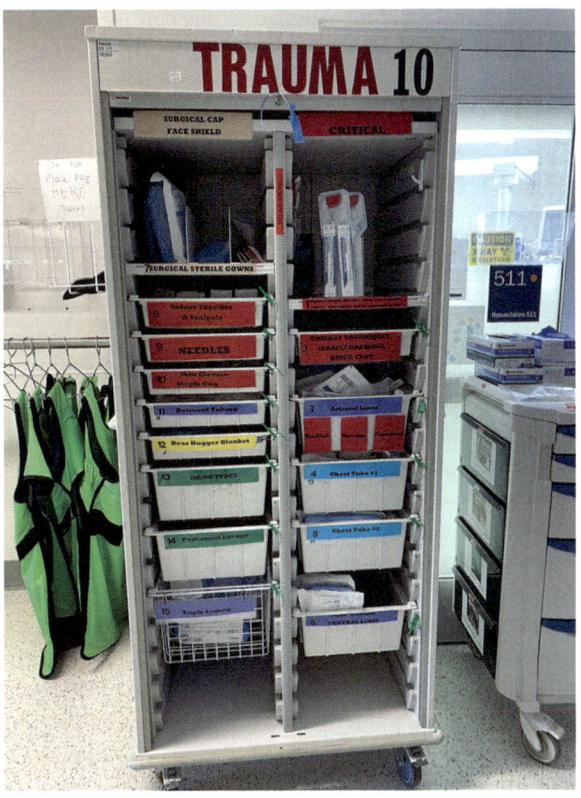

From my extensive experience doing site visits, I have seen many innovative equipment solutions. This included placing a cutting shear on a retractable string hanging over the trauma bay that was replaced after each use, taping scalpers to the closest wall to the stretcher, intubation equipment rolls, anesthesia machines in the trauma bat, and many others. Innovative equipment solutions can streamline resuscitations and avoid conflicts and frustration. It is important for any trauma program to take equipment opportunities seriously and devote sufficient effort to correct them and improve care.

Guidelines

Guideline creation dissemination and enforcement are probably the most complex and time-consuming activities that the PI program can undertake. However, guidelines are without question the most effective way to decrease variation in care and improved outcomes. "If there are 10 different ways to do something, then it's unlikely that any of them are the best". Even if there were 10 completely equivalent ways to handle a clinical situation, the confusion that would be caused by having 10 physicians handle the same problem in 10 different ways would likely offset any benefit.

It is important to remember that guidelines are merely a tool to measure variation. If you do not have a guideline, then you have no way of examining the processes of care and looking at consistent decision-making. Guidelines should not be viewed as laws because they often have to be changed and adapted as new evidence presents itself, or if after implementation it is obvious that the guideline is making things worse. What I have often said is the guidelines provide you a tool that codifies experience. So instead of having active follow around senior clinicians to learn how to do things, a group of senior clinicians can get together and examine the evidence and put together tools that anyone can use it any time of day to avoid improvisation.

Guidelines are not a ubiquitous tool in PI. Creating a guideline for every situation would probably lead people to ignore them. You need to focus your efforts on those clinical situations where the risk of patient harm is high, where the cost of improvisation is high, or where the nature of the clinical situation demands that everyone be on the same page rapidly to avoid mayhem. I have published guidelines for trauma center since my arrival in June 1994. These guidelines were originally on paper and then were converted into a spiral-bound pocket guide, and then are in its present form which is an application that can be downloaded onto an iPhone or any other handheld device. While I examine the evidence and created the guideline in 1994 by myself, guidelines have become a completely collaborative effort in 2020. Guidelines related to specific specialties are vetted by our liaisons in the specialties, and guidelines related to the trauma service are created by a small group pass through the medical director and then through the acute care surgery faculty for comment until they are finally published.

Guidelines are most useful in loop closure when you encounter opportunities for improvement in situations that are relatively common (e.g., splenic injury), or where there is no good evidence for one process over another. (Clearance of the cervical spine using CT scan). For the latter example, you can still get a group of trauma surgeons together to discuss this issue and get several different ways of doing things. Not only does this lead to variation and the potential for confusion and adverse clinical outcomes, but it does not provide a consistent way to address this issue that other staff and learners can use. Also in that latter example your group needs to look at the evidence and come up with the guideline that captures as much of the evidence as possible. I believe this is an important point in that if you create a guideline that is based on flimsy evidence, or which was created without some sort of consensus it will almost certainly fail. Creating guidelines without input from multiple sources, or creating a guideline without bringing detractors into the tent, will lead to sabotage. People will criticize the guideline, say that they were not involved in its creation, and that it will not be followed. In those situations, guidelines are almost useless.

However, you are often not going to be able to get all stakeholders to agree. This is where a trauma medical director needs some talent in being able to bring a group of people together, even people who are difficult, and bring them to a reasonable consensus on how to treat patients. This is often easier in an academic setting where clinicians are usually more cognizant of the current evidence and where care is usually provided in a team like structure, that it might be in some community hospitals where every clinician practices independent of every other. It is important for the trauma medical director to show a willingness to compromise if a faction is extremely critical of certain aspects of the guideline and possibly create a guideline that may not be 100% evidence-based but which will improve care and decrease variation.

Probably the most common guidelines for trauma centers are those for spine clearance. Most trauma programs have instances where someone had spinal precautions removed too early and may have suffered exacerbation of an injury, or someone whose spinal precautions were longer than necessary to develop the pressure ulcers. There is quite a bit of evidence for spine clearance, but some of it is contradictory. Also the trauma service usually has a philosophy that they are going to be more paranoid about the possibility of missing a critical injury then perhaps in emergency medicine physician. This is out of necessity since an emergency medicine physician is usually facing a large number of patients every day with minimal injuries who cannot go through an extensive radiological workup and must have process that uses criteria that may be somewhat more liberal than an acute-care surgeon taking care of multiple trauma patient. This is not being that the emergency medicine physician is practicing credit medicine incorrectly, it only means that in an emergency room the evidence may be interpreted in such a way to allow leeway in using clinician judgment to clear the spine. However, there are always instances where an aggressive philosophy toward clearing the spines may discharge a patient with an injury who would then return and thus go through the trauma PI process.

The usual process is to move from a case that demonstrates an opportunity for improvement, to the analysis of the issue and the suggestion that a guideline in this clinical situation would be appropriate. Then a group of clinicians should be tasked with examining the evidence and creating a draft guideline. In our institution, these draft guidelines are presented at our multidisciplinary PI meeting for input and are sent out to all of the liaisons for comment. We have also tried to obtain guidelines for similar issues from other institutions and incorporated their creations into ours. There is no reason to reinvent the wheel in every situation. If another trauma center has spent the time and effort to develop clinical practice guidelines that encompasses all available clinical evidence it should be replicated in your program. Of course you need to give attribution to the center that created the guideline.

Guidelines should be simple to read and should guide the reader quickly through the steps. We have always used flowcharts to do this as this is the most common way to represent the process of clinical practice. However there are some guidelines that can be written in prose, or with bullet points depending on the nature of the situation you are trying to address. Once the guideline has been approved by consensus, you must undertake an education plan. Usually just sending an email to clinicians with an attachment will not be successful. In academic centers, specific education to residents and advanced practice practitioners regarding the guidelines necessary. And of course examining the clinical process corralled by the guideline going forward is necessary in some extent to ensure that the guideline is being affected. If you find that the same PI issues and it recurs even after guidelines been disseminated and is in place for a reasonable period of time, there needs to be a postmortem of the event and the guideline to try to understand why it was followed. In most instances, guideline deviance occurs in the middle of the night, with new practitioners, or in situations where the clinical issue is misdiagnosed or unappreciated.

Site visit teams love the institution of guidelines and that demonstrates that the PI program is willing to extend significant effort to address an opportunity for improvement. For us, creation and implementation of the guideline is in some ways the gold standard for PI activities. However, we are well aware that guidelines can be published and never followed. We will often ask the program to provide a summary of whether the opportunity addressed by the guideline has recurred, and how they know that guideline is actually being followed. This does not need to be perfect but merely needs to recognize that simply emailing guidelines to people does not ensure the clinical practice will change. We also give significant credit the creation of a guideline that may have difficulty in implementation. Also remember site visit teams are usually seen by your trauma medical directors that have been through this and can provide advice as to how to create more interference to a clinical practice guideline. A final thought on this matter is that some hospitals have different names for guidelines and depending on what name you attached for what you have created will be the amount of aggravation you will need to go through to get it published and implemented. In some centers, clinical guidelines can be interpreted as "policies." Obviously, the process for the implementation of the policies is far different than an educational guide. Policies usually need to be vetted at multiple levels of hospital administration and often need to be improved by practice committees. These committees often have very little to no knowledge of the clinical situation that the trauma service faces and can insert unnecessary delay in implementation. This is why it is important for you to understand how your hospital views these sorts of activities. In our hospital, calling something a clinical practice guideline creates a fairly simple path to publishing; however, it does require that the guideline be reevaluated at some yearly interval and updated as new evidence emerges. This is a reasonable requirement for any guideline.

After site visit, any guideline should be presented to the team along with the opportunity for improvement that instigated it, how you created, and then how you implemented at audit. Since many guidelines are not attached to a single case, I feel the process of aggregating the same opportunity across multiple cases into a PI project that then leads to a guideline is an excellent way to organize this activity. Our UVA trauma center guidelines are available online at http://www.healthsystem. virginia.edu/pub/trauma-center/2015TraumaManual364599_Final_.pdf

Hardwiring Change

Hardwired and change in a trauma center can be very difficult and frustrating. There are always new clinicians starting their jobs and experienced clinicians retiring and moving on to other facilities. There can be changes in management of unit as well as changes in leadership. Thus the trauma program should develop a process by which they try to ensure as much as possible that optimal care is provided.

Use of EMR

Use of an electronic medical record is probably the easiest and most effective way to control variation in practice and implement new measures. In most facilities, now orders cannot be placed outside of the electronic medical record and electronic ordering system. Thus, hard stops and advisories can flash on the screen. When certain criteria are met by the provider, it can be extremely useful. Since you must always have the option for the provider to disregard advisories (because there are instances where it is incorrectly applied), it is possible for providers to bypass any action you put in to control variation. This is why consensus is so important in that hostility toward an effort to rein in clinical practice can always sabotage the effort.

While I will not mention any vendors for electronic medical records, here it was well known to programs that some vendors provide an easy way to change ordering pathways and advisories and some have such an onerous method for re-coding their software that it is almost futile. It is important for the PI staff to learn what is needed to change the electronic software to provide recommendations or guide clinicians down a certain pathway. While this is the most effective way to implement change, it is probably the most difficult depending on the electronic medical records you have in place. In addition, some electronic systems do not really provide a method for controlling clinical variation. In those cases, and even if your medic goal record has a way to implement change, posters, welcome screen advisories, applications, can all also be very effective. In the trauma bay, large posters indicating clinical guidelines can be extremely effective in that it is unlikely that someone is to pull out their phone and open an application, or go through their email in the midst of her resuscitation. Obviously you cannot have the walls of the resuscitation bay papered with posters, but three or four key processes can usually be placed unobtrusively. In addition, new protocols can be given the space to try to improve implementation.

Gatekeepers and Safety Officers

When implementing guidelines or procedural standard work, it is necessary to have someone who can monitor the process. If you do not provide some monitoring of these processes, then the only way you can know if they were affected was by looking at outcome. But as we all know most measures will not significantly affect outcomes but will merely refine and improve the process of care. If a center implemented a loop closure tool that significantly decreased their mortality, I would be very worried about the care that that center was providing before we implemented the process. There are some adverse events such as ventilator-associated pneumonia, central line-associated bloodstream infection, and catheter-associated urinary tract infection which may share significant change after implementation of improvement. Thankfully most of these outcome measures are measured by the hospital quality program and do not need to be measured by the trauma program. Once again, it is essential that the trauma program and the hospital quality program be integrated and share information.

For standard work in emergency department and intensive care unit, it is often difficult to implement auditing all hours of the day. In addition, in my experience, nurses tend to be generally uncomfortable with being the "patient police" and calling out deviations from standard methods. However there really is no one as well-placed as the bedside nurse to know if guidelines were followed and standard work was used. Asking nurses to monitor these processes will usually require compromise and a method by which the nurse does not need to directly confront the offender. This can include what we have used in our institution where as the nurses are empowered to send an email to the trauma director or the trauma program manager to report a problem and then the trauma program should go about correction.

At this point, I would like to interject the process I have used for many years to corral physician behavior. When a deviation from standard work is reported or observed by the physician, it is for the most part unlikely that that was the only instance of deviation. If you can be sure that that single clinician is the sole person who is not following standard work, then a one-on-one intervention is appropriate. However in the thousands of times I have tried that it usually turns into a "he said she said" situation and nothing usually gets done. What I have done that is worked very well is to send communication to all the relevant clinicians who are supposed to follow the standard work reiterating that we all agreed that this was going to be our process and that if you do not want to follow the process do not simply ignore it but come to the committees and explain your aversion and suggest an improvement. What I have often found is that people who were following standard work immediately email me and say "was this me?" I feel that this somewhat general loop closure and intervention tends to keep people from being defensive, and also serves the purpose of reiterating a loop closure process to the entire group further reinforcing it.

Your trauma registry can play a role in auditing standard work; however, most registry programs are understaffed and with the addition of TQIP data extraction to their normal extraction duties, there is usually insufficient and with two audit charts for standard work. But for outcomes that are routinely extracted, registry queries can be very useful in monitoring loop closure. For instance, if you adapt your non-operative splenic management protocol to indicate that patients with grade 1 and grade 2 injuries should not be over 24 hours if the blood counts are stable, it is easy for a registrar to pull patient's records with this injury and their length of stay. Of course, there may be other injuries that forced a longer admission, but the registrar should also be able to provide that additional information. Another question arises as to whether you should add fields your registry as loop closure is implemented for monitoring. You need to be somewhat careful about this or your registry will expand by dozens of fields causing problems of its own. We usually opt not adding additional fields but designing reports that pull from already abstracted data to help us audit loop closure. It is not wrong to add fields for a short period of time and then remove them, but some registries make this a little difficult. As far as integrating with your electronic medical record to audit loop closure, this would absolutely depend on your vendor and your ability to modify your products. In general, the engineers can modify the electronic medical record, are usually overwhelmed with requests, and there will, almost certainly, be a delay in implementing change if that occurs at all.

Audits do not need to continue ad infinitum. When you discuss loop closure implementation, you should first determine how long you will monitor the process. If it is a process that occurs regularly, 3 months may be sufficient; if it is a process that occurs rarely, a year may be required. But if every loop closure is monitored forever, you will soon run out of bandwidth to monitor anything else of importance. Site viewers will not object to a limited monitoring period as long as you demonstrate compliance. If at the end of your monitoring you cannot prove compliance with the new measures, you would have to provide an explanation as to why you were abandoning this loop closure product, or demonstrate the discussion at your meetings where the unsatisfactory results were presented and corrective measures were suggested and implemented.

As I said previously loop closure is probably the single most important part of performance improvement. You must design your loop closure efforts carefully, try as best you can to integrate them into already existing standard work, and provide some ability to monitor compliance with the new process, for the site visit documentation is key. Make sure that you clearly document the opportunity, the rationale for the loop closure product, the methods that you undertook to implement, and auditing and results. I also believe it is far easier to aggregate multiple cases with the same problem into a single project.

Chapter 11
Types of Issues

In this chapter we begin the discussion of specific and common areas of performance improvement investigation. There will be more extensive case studies in the final part of this book. In this chapter, we present small vignettes of the cases to represent the issues involved.

Clinician Performance and Decision-Making

We are going to start with the hardest issue first. Dealing with subpar clinical performance and decision-making can be the most difficult PI problem to correct. As we all know, medical decision-making is not always guided by evidence and that other factors can often play a role. Some clinicians are very focused on cost containment which will sway them against extensive testing. While others may be hyper-aggressive toward low-risk problems creating their own set of issues.

Vignette 1

A 24-year-old male arrived at the emergency after falling off an all-terrain vehicle. The EMS report indicates that the patient is found awake and complaining of right thigh pain and left-sided chest pain. The patient's vital signs were normal, and the patient was awake and oriented. The emergency department performs a chest X-ray that shows several rib fractures and no evidence of pneumothorax, and a pelvic X-ray that is negative for injury. A right thigh X-ray demonstrates a mid-shaft right femur fracture. Orthopedics is called to evaluate the patient and they request a trauma evaluation. The on-call trauma attending comes down to see the patient and finds that the vital signs are stable, the patient is awake, and is complaining of

J. S. Young, *Trauma Center Performance Improvement*,
https://doi.org/10.1007/978-3-030-71048-4_11

left-sided chest pain and right thigh pain. The trauma attending performs a fast exam which is equivocal for fluid in the pelvis. The attending indicates in their note that they felt that the abdomen was benign except for some pain in the left upper quadrant that they attributed to the rib fractures. The trauma attending approved the orthopedic plan to take the patient to the operating room and fix the femur fracture. At this point, laboratory values come back and the patient's lactic acid is 2.8. No further workup is performed.

The patient is taken to the operating room for the fixation of the right femur and 1 hour into the case becomes hypotensive. The trauma attending is called to the operating room and finds that the patient's blood pressure is 60/40 and his pulse rate is 130. He talked to the orthopedic surgeons who indicate that they have not had any significant blood loss at this point. The patient is given 4 liters of fluid and blood is ordered. The patient continues to do poorly and is refractory to these measures. The patient's abdomen appears to be distending, and the trauma attending elects to perform laparoscopy. It takes approximately 20 minutes to set up for laparoscopy, and upon inserting the trocar in the abdomen, the patient suffered a cardiac arrest. The abdomen is rapidly opened and 4 liters of blood is found along with an actively bleeding grade IV splenic injury. The patient is resuscitated and taken to the surgical intensive care unit but suffers multiple organ failure and dies several days later.

Performance Improvement Investigation

The case is identified the following morning, and the PI program was notified of the mortality. The PI coordinator goes through the patient record and contacts the trauma medical director due to their immediate opinion that this is a preventable death and requires urgent analysis. The initial analysis of the case finds several opportunities for improvement of which the most important is an inadequate workup in the emergency department. This trauma program does not have widely distributed guidelines for the routine workup of the trauma patient. As a community hospital, the trauma surgeons are staffed by one fellowship-trained surgeon and six community general surgeons. The community general surgeons have obstructed the implementation of guidelines saying that every patient is different and that there is no rational way to treat all patients the same.

To document the process up to this point, an initial abstraction of the chart should be completed and placed in the trauma PI program records to indicate that there was rapid examination of the case.

The trauma medical director contacts the original attending surgeon and discusses the case. The treating attending reinforces the written record that the patient's abdomen was essentially benign and they felt that cross-sectional imaging was not warranted. They did not perform an ultrasound exam because they felt that in their hands it was inaccurate, and they did not ask the emergency physician to perform one.

Discussion

This is perhaps the most frightening example of the danger of excessive variability in a trauma center. While many physicians will balk at the idea of performing a set group of tests in each trauma patient that demonstrates a significant mechanism of injury, there has been a fair amount of scientific evidence that the physical exam is untrustworthy when it comes to evaluating for fluid in the abdomen, that observing the patient for several hours can in some cases substitute for imaging but is still not 100% accurate, and that mechanism of injury is not a valid way to determine that a trauma patient is at risk for serious injury.

In this case, the fact that the patient had a femur fracture on one side and chest injuries on the opposite side and that they were in a vehicle where it was likely that they could not remain in the seat, and were ejected during the accident should have prompted the emergency room physician and the trauma surgeon to carry out a more thorough workup. In addition, the evidence of a mid-shaft femur fracture indicates that there was a fair amount of force transmitted to the patient. The equivocal ultrasound exam also should have raised concerns for the attending surgeon. It is reasonable to expect that had cross-sectional imaging been performed, the splenic laceration would have been identified. It is also reasonable to expect that since the patient degenerated quickly, extravasation would have been demonstrated on the scan. At that point, the patient could have been taken to angiography prior to orthopedic surgery or the operating room for exploration prior to femur fixation. Doing either of these would have saved the patient's life.

At this point, the trauma medical director is faced with several hard choices. This is an unexpected death with several opportunities for improvement and reflects badly on the trauma center's performance and upon the surgeon involved. However, it is difficult to control surgical judgment in all situations and at all times of day. The surgeon's reasoning may appear flawed to the medical director, but it may appear reasonable for the other members of the trauma panel. Another factor which should be included in the investigation is whether cases like this had happened before for this physician. Assuming there had not been any previous cases such as this, the most effective corrective action would be a thorough discussion of the case at the PI meeting with all of the attending surgeons present. The trauma medical director should be prepared with evidence from the literature that findings indicating a high level of force transmitted to a patient as evidenced by the femur fracture and injuries on the contralateral side of the body warrant cross-sectional imaging. There may be disagreement, but it is the job of the trauma medical director to steer the conversation toward what is safest for the patient. This is especially important in those cases where the patient will be unable to be examined for several hours because of orthopedic procedures. As we know, in the operating room transient hypotension could be attributed to non-bleeding causes and can often be treated with blood pressure–elevating medications. This will mask bleeding and make the situation worse. Thus, it is imperative to identify potential sources of bleeding before a patient is taken for orthopedic procedures. The easiest way to do this is to obtain cross-sectional imaging of the chest, abdomen, and pelvis. If this is an American College of

Surgeons–verified center, consistency in the evaluation of the injured patient and minimization of variability are very important to the site visitors. A case such as this, where an unexpected death occurred from a readily treatable injury will be examined extremely closely and a robust corrective action plan will be expected. It should be noted that when there is consistency in the workup of these patients, time spent getting imaging can be minimized since the emergency department can begin imaging immediately if the trauma center has consistent guidelines for the diagnostic evaluation. It should also be emphasized that the physical exam is notoriously unreliable in ruling out abdominal injuries, especially solid organ injuries. It should also be noted that the patient did demonstrate physical signs and symptoms that could certainly demonstrate a splenic injury since the patient had tenderness on the left side of the chest and complained of pain in the left chest and left upper quadrant.

Corrective Action Plan

If this surgeon had had a history of similar lapses in judgment, reporting up the hierarchy about concerns for the surgeon's ability to properly function on the trauma panel should be considered. However if there is overall a great degree of variability in your program, this attending surgeon cannot really be blamed for this entire outcome. It is in some ways the fault of the program to allow a great deal of latitude in how patients are evaluated. There should certainly be a personal discussion with the attending surgeon about this case with the trauma medical director and this should be documented. Below is an example of the documentation to put in the PI records:

> I discussed the case of MRN 1123345 with Dr Smith on September 3, 2020, at 4 PM. We reviewed the details of the case and I expressed my concerns with the patient's management. Dr Smith indicated that he felt that the clinical evaluation did not warrant a complete radiologic evaluation; however, in light of this case he would follow any guidelines that were created to decrease variability in the case of these patients.

However the discussion at the PI meeting with consensus about the creation of a consistent standard for diagnostic evaluation for patients with severe mechanisms of injury, or with certain types of injuries, will be a far more effective loop closure. When creating new guidelines, the program should not reinvent the wheel and should contact mature programs to see if they have similar guidelines. Even if their guidelines are not appropriate for your center, it will provide a template for your guideline.

Blood Transfusion Error

Vignette #2

A 41-year-old female patient presents to the emergency department after a motor vehicle crash. The patient is hypotensive on arrival but awake and oriented. Chest X-ray Is normal, and the patient has a minor pubic fracture. The patient is given 2 liters of crystalloid, and an ultrasound (FAST) exam reveals blood in all quadrants. The patient is given two units of blood from the emergency department refrigerator, but her blood pressure stays below 90. The patient is taken in the operating room.

The patient is hypotensive with blood pressures of 80/60 despite blood transfusion and the operation begins. The surgeon rapidly controls the splenic hilum after finding a shattered spleen and finds about 1.5 L of blood in the abdomen. The surgeon tells the anesthesiologist that they think they have things under control and the patient just needs be resuscitated. The type and crossmatched blood is delivered to the operating room. Unbeknownst to the surgical team, the anesthesiologist felt that they could not take sufficient time to do all of the checks required before administering the blood because they felt the patient was grossly unstable. She begins to hang a unit from the cooler and the patient becomes tachycardic and their temperature begins to rise. The transfusion is stopped and the bag is sequestered and it is elected to wait for type and crossmatched blood. The operation ends and the patient recovers uneventfully.

Performance Improvement Investigation

A quality report is automatically generated for suspected blood transfusion reaction. Blood is drawn from the patient and the unit of blood is sent to the blood bank. Later that day, it is found that there was an ABO incompatibility between the blood that was administered (blood was A, patient was B). Additional labs are sent and the patient has a small bump in her creatinine but otherwise no ill effects of the transfusion. The attending physician and the blood bank Fellow inform the patient and their family of the error (by hospital policy, the anesthesiologist is not required to be part of the conversation). Since there was no significant sequelae, the patient and the family thanked the team for saving her life.

Investigation reveals that while this patient was going up to the operating room, another anonymous trauma patient had been alerted. This patient also had type and crossmatched blood, but the process was several minutes behind the patient with the spleen injury. However, both patients had trauma numbers that are provided for anonymous patients. At this time, the numbers have the format T9012345, and the first four letters of the last name were added to the end of the record number after their identification was confirmed (i.e., T9012345SMIT). However, at this time, only the seven-digit number was available. The spleen patient's number was T9015432, and the other patient's number was T9015433. At this time, consecutive unknown patients were given consecutive numbers. The transporter who was bringing the blood from the blood bank asked the charge nurse where the trauma patient was and was directed to the room where the laparotomy was being performed. The transporter left the blood cooler with the anesthesiologist. Instead of doing all the checks required the anesthesiologist merely looked at the units and saw that it was a trauma number and administered the blood. The root cause for the error was actually found toward the latter portion of the case when the blood for the second trauma patient never arrived in the operating room when the second patient was in, and the blood bank was called and they stated that a cooler was sent 30 minutes previously. The OR quickly identified what was going on and informed the blood bank.

Discussion

Obviously, there was a significant provider error in this case. Even if the patient had been grossly hypotensive, which they were not, it would not have been acceptable for the anesthesiologist to bypass the safety checks. The hospital at this time did not yet have a barcoding system on the patient's ID so safety checks required manually reading the patient's number off of a risk label and comparing it to the blood. Another problem in acute trauma patients is that often the wristband is not accessible due to draping in other factors, and anesthesiologists often cut off the wristband and tape it to the anesthesia machine in these cases.

There were several opportunities for improvement: the provider error, the method and process for checking the blood, the transporter's error in delivering the blood to the wrong room, the ambiguous naming system for anonymous trauma patients, and the communication between the surgeon and the anesthesiologist.

Corrective Actions

The corrective action involving the provider was fairly straightforward. The anesthesiologist liaison was contacted as well is the chair of the department. The details of the event were described and they were asked to discuss this directly with the anesthesiologist involved. This conversation was documented through an email and placed in the PI records. It was felt by the trauma team that it was inappropriate for the trauma attending to be required to inform the patient and family of this error when the person who had made the mistake is not required to talk to the patient and the family. This was part of the hospital policy that stated that the attending physician is ultimately responsible for these communications and did not directly require any other faculty involved. This was brought up with the hospital quality committee, and the policy was amended to require the attending physician and any physician who was involved in the error. This policy was approved as loop closure on this small issue.

The trauma program was not completely satisfied with the corrective action regarding the anesthesiologists. This was felt to be a very, very serious error and more than a discussion should have occurred. The trauma medical director discussed this with the anesthesia department, but the anesthesiologist involved in the case simply felt that the patient was dying and that the safety checks needed to be bypassed. In light of this it was agreed that the anesthesiologists' practice should be audited for a year and the quality officer of the hospital and the credentials commit-tee were informed of the error and the plan for continued monitoring. This is an example that sometimes the trauma program cannot get everything it wants but must compromise.

It was felt the method and process used for checking blood in the operating room was not optimal. It required a clinician whose attention was being drawn in several directions with a critical patient to try to concentrate on checking the blood when they had several other tasks that needed to be performed simultaneously. While it was common for additional anesthesia help to be called into these cases, this was made part of policy after this case. At least two anesthesiologists had to be assigned to the case until the patient had stabilized, or an anesthesiologist and a nurse anes-thetist could suffice. In addition, an anesthesia technician would be assigned to these cases, as their sole task, until the patient was stable. This was also the case that further pushed the hospital toward implementing barcoding on patient's wristbands and on medications and blood as another high-level safety check to prevent error. The loop closure was documented as the change in the classroom for anesthesia during these cases, and the implementation of barcoding as a safety measure.

The issue with the transporter was actually found to be a significant issue throughout the hospital. In querying the ICU, an additional potential for error was found in that blood was often placed in the pneumatic tubes and sent to the unit without a double check at the tube station. It was found from looking back at several safety reports that the patient care assistant in the ICU would be told blood is being sent up from the blood bank and would rush over to the tube station, grab it, and bring it to the room. It was found there were several near misses where a clini-cian brought the blood to the wrong room. This often occured when there was more than one critically ill patient receiving blood (which is common in surgical ICUs). Therefore, in addition to barcoding, an extra step in the process was made that a nurse would have to pick up the blood at the tube station and do an immediate check with the information from the patient who was to receive the blood. It was then implemented that there will be another check at the door to the room so that the blood would not get into the room until two safety checks were done. This was implemented and documented as loop closure.

Staffing and Education Problems

Vignette #3

A 75-year-old patient is being treated in the trauma intensive care unit for multiple orthopedic fractures, pulmonary contusion, grade I splenic injury, and mild head injury. The patient is intubated but hemodynamically stable. That night several criti-cal trauma patients were admitted, and the nurse caring for this patient was also caring for another trauma patient in the ICU. During the night, this patient began to exhibit some hemodynamic instability. There was a first postgraduate year resident staffing the trauma ICU during this shift. The patient's blood pressure had dropped to 100/60. The patient had a norepinephrine drip hanging by the bedside for the past 24 hours following an incident when the patient was given excessive sedation for an orthopedic manipulation and became hypotensive. Since there was no evidence of bleeding, a short-term course of norepinephrine was used and then stopped approximately (8 hours previously). The nurse hooks up the norepinephrine drip and increases the rate. The patient is now on 4 micrograms of norepinephrine and their blood pressure is still 90/60. At this point, the nurse contacts the resident in the ICU who orders a 2 L normal saline bolus. After the 2 L bolus and raising the norepinephrine drip to 8, the patient's hypotension persists. The resident raises a norepinephrine drip to 12 and orders another 2 L bolus. After 90 minutes of this, the charge nurse walks by the room, sees what is going on, and immediately contacts the chief resident. The chief resident arrives and after assessing the situation orders labs, a chest X-ray, EKG, and performs a physical exam. The patient's abdomen is slightly more distended than previously and the chief resident brings an ultrasound machine to the bedside and finds fluid throughout the abdomen. When the labs return, the patient's hemoglobin has dropped by 40%. At this point, the patient begins to have some cardiac irregularities and goes into atrial fibrillation. This further worsens the patient's hypotension. The chief resident notifies the attending trauma surgeon and immediately calls for three units of blood, plasma, and emergency CT scan of the abdomen. After giving the blood, they are able to decrease the norepinephrine dose, but the patient's lactic acid is 8.5. The CT scan shows a marked increase in fluid in the abdomen and what appears to be a ruptured subcapsular hematoma of the spleen with active extravasation. Due to the patient's instability, they are rushed to the operating room where splenectomy is performed. Postoperatively the patient goes into renal failure, has long-standing respiratory failure requiring tracheostomy, and has bouts of multiple infections. The patient is eventually discharged to a skilled nursing facility.

Performance Improvement

The case is identified by the charge nurse in the ICU with regard to the resident performance and the chief resident with regard to the nursing performance. One thing to mention at this point is that this patient did not die, and this is a great example of how important it is to have surveillance for OFIs well beyond just mortality. Clearly this patient's care was suboptimal, and there are many opportunities for improvement. But in some programs, because the patient did not die, this case would not have a high priority. In addition, the patient's age and multiple injuries may lead the program to believe that this would not be an unexpected death had that occurred. It is very important to separate the risk of mortality to the patient based on their age, injuries, and comorbidities, and the presence of opportunities for improvement that may or may not have impacted the patient's outcome but may impact future patients. This case is an excellent example of multiple opportunities for improvement that need to be addressed.

Analysis and Opportunities for Improvement

There are several opportunities for improvement in this case. First, is the proper identification and treatment of hypotension, bleeding, and possible sepsis in the intensive care unit. Trauma patients may often be hemodynamically stable for extended periods of time even though they have several critical injuries. As we like to say "the only certainty in life is that things change and life is dynamic." The patient's previous 48 hours of stability does not guarantee that that condition will persist in the next hour.

In any fresh trauma patient, or even a trauma patient several days out, hypotension that does not respond rapidly to a simple intervention should be considered to be a critical sign of bleeding. As time from admission extends, the risk of bleeding decreases and the risk of sepsis increases.

In order to intervene effectively in patients with sepsis, you must identify the condition, initiate rapid treatment including resuscitation, source control, and targeted antibiotic therapy.

To intervene effectively for bleeding, you must first rapidly resuscitate the patient meaning that you have to have sufficient intravenous access, blood available, and try to avoid the use of vasopressor agents since they can mask a worsening hemodynamic condition. Once the patient is stable enough for transport, cavitary scanning is necessary to identify the source of bleeding, unless there is a strong suspicion from previous studies as to the source of bleeding. In that case, the patient can be taken directly for intervention in the OR or interventional radiology suite. A chest X-ray should be rapidly obtained in the ICU before leaving the ICU to ensure that there are no sources of bleeding in the chest. If a critical source of bleeding is identified that requires operative intervention, the trauma center must be able to find an operating room and team within 30 minutes 24 hours a day.

After doing this, it is critical to closely observe the patient for response to therapy and initiate further treatments should they be necessary.

Second is communication between providers. A system was already in place in this intensive care unit to bring experienced help to the bedside rapidly. This institution had an in-house intensivist/trauma surgeon readily available to respond if needed. However, any backup safety system is of no use if it is not activated. In order for a safety system to be activated, the frontline providers must realize that they are in a situation that requires expertise that they do not possess. There are many ways to create a system where expertise is brought to the bedside automatically, but all of these systems have drawbacks. A proper sign-out system is critical between and among nurses and physicians in order to ensure that the oncoming team is cognizant of the risks to the patient during their shift. This includes respiratory decompensation, hemodynamic decompensation, risk of infection, agitation, and risk of declining mental status. However, patients' conditions are dynamic and even the best sign-out will not anticipate problems that arise during a shift. Also, realistically, if an oncoming resident is covering a large number of patients, no sign-out will provide sufficient information for complex issues that arise in a patient. The resident will need to get up and go see the patient, examine them, read the chart, discuss the condition with the nurses, and formulate a plan.

Finally, a vexing problem is the fear of escalation for inexperienced residents. This fear is a result of criticism of previous escalations, or simply a poor relationship between the frontline resident and their supervising resident or attending. It is a fairly common problem in both community hospitals and academic medical centers where a junior employee or resident is fearful of escalating above the clinician that they are working with. Obviously this can be detrimental to a relationship for a nurse to disregard what the physician in the room is saying and go to their superior, but the first priority needs to be the patient's health. In our own institution, the creation of a rapid response team exemplified these problems. Though we created hard activation triggers for calling the team, we found that in many instances, the intern or second-year resident at the bedside would tell the nurse not to activate the team. After several very adverse outcomes and deaths from a lack of escalation, and the lack of activating an infrastructure created solely for the purpose of intervening in critical situations, we as a medical center took a hard line toward these actions. We instructed all residents, nurse practitioners, physician assistants, and clinicians that if it was reported to us that the patient met activation triggers for the rapid response team and the team was not called because someone said they should not be called these could potentially be firing offenses and/or a credentialing issue. After instituting this policy, these instances decreased significantly, but we still monitor these activations closely because it is easy for problems to creep back in whenever inexperienced and insecure providers begin taking care of patients. In this case, it is unclear whether this was the problem, for the trauma program must always entertain that there was fear of escalation in situations such as this and to provide support to the nurse at the bedside or whatever clinician is at the bedside, to make them understand that putting the patient first will always be defensible. If in this case it was identified that there was a problem with fear of escalation, then the clinician who prevented escalation should be personally spoken with by either the trauma director or the specialty liaisons, or if under the purview of nursing, the chief nursing officer to instruct them that is always a better practice to allow escalation to occur rather than to stop it and place the burden for any problems the patient may have on their head.

External Issues (EMS, Transfer Hospitals)

Vignette #4

Next, we will turn to the issues that are external to the trauma center which include problems with EMS, and with transferring hospitals. First, we will discuss EMS.

I have extensive experience with EMS agencies and am currently an operational medical director for several. In addition, I practiced as a medic for several years during college and medical school with several agencies, so I do understand the issues that street providers face. Where these issues interact with the trauma center often revolve around failure to recognize the dire condition of the patient, recognize the condition of the patient but not appropriately activating aeromedical transport to get the patient to the nearest trauma center as quickly as possible, or taking the patient to the nearest hospital that is not a trauma center when the difference in time between transporting to the nearest hospital versus the trauma center was small enough to make the decision unwise.

In most jurisdictions, EMS can be controlled by the local government, a private agency, local fire departments, volunteers, career personnel, or hospitals. I have seen EMS systems controlled by each of these entities in my experience with site visits. There is no one administrative process that is better than any other. While many of us would prefer that the medics we deal with are career employees and not part-time volunteers, there are volunteer agencies that provide exemplary care and care that often will exceed that provided by paid providers. What is essential to good patient care is the involvement of the operational medical director, a good performance improvement process within the agency, closed-loop communication between the trauma center and the agency, and a willingness on both sides to adapt to circumstances.

Another issue that often plagues trauma centers is the lack of adequate warning of the arrival of a critical trauma patient. This can be unavoidable in certain jurisdictions (e.g., New York City) where travel times may be very short, especially when the trauma patient is injured within several blocks of the hospital. But even in those jurisdictions, 911 centers can set up processes by which they inform the trauma center emergency department that they have dispatched the unit for a potentially critically ill trauma patient. Also, some jurisdictions have gone to voice-activated headsets and/or Bluetooth earpieces that allow them to continue to provide care and move the patient toward the hospital while providing some information to the receiving facility. It is critical to not simply criticize these agencies when they do not provide adequate warning. You must demonstrate to them that no trauma center can have a trauma team waiting in the resuscitation bay at all hours of the day. It takes time to assemble the team, assemble equipment, and brief the team in preparation for the arrival of a critically ill trauma patient. The trauma center should endeavor to keep this time short (less than 10 minutes), and there should be contingency plans to bring clinicians to the bedside rapidly should a patient arrive unannounced as they do in major urban areas. But through our own performance improvement process, and that of centers I reviewed, when the patient arrives without warning, the trauma team is often behind the curve. They are reacting to circumstances as they encounter them, after the patient has already been in the emergency department for several minutes and care can be disjointed and sometimes dangerous. A common root cause we have found in these situations is inadequate warning to allow the trauma center to take the time necessary to prepare itself optimally for patient arrival. Regarding this PI problem, we have communicated directly to agencies, provided lectures to these agencies about the trauma activation process, worked with these agencies to help them understand our activation criteria, had medics rotate with our trauma service and in our emergency department to better understand the process of trauma activation, and put in place protocols and guidelines by which the 911 center or dispatching personnel can notify the hospital without burdening the street team. There will always be instances where warning will be inadequate, but the center should audit this and if it occurs repeatedly and warning is possible, they should work with the EMS agency to improve performance.

Every ACS site visit asks about the process where EMS agencies are provided feedback and how PI problems are investigated and closed. There are many ways to do this: having a Fire/ EMS officer on the PI committee, developing relationships with the operational medical director and chief of these agencies, working with local or regional EMS councils to provide feedback to individual agencies, and or creating protocols and guidelines to help field providers provide the best care possible. I have found that providing educational opportunities to agencies about what we actually do in a trauma center opens their eyes to the importance of the care that they provide. A common issue is intubation. Rapid sequence intubation is becoming less and less common throughout the United States with some studies showing that the average paramedic does between one and two of these every year on actual patients, and often this is in a cardiac arrest. It has been well demonstrated that the volume of intubations a medic does improves their performance. If a missed inhibition is identified, it invariably contributes to mortality and warrants investigation. The trauma center PI group should work with the EMS agency to quickly gather the facts and query an administrative officer from the agency about the circumstances of the call. They should focus on whether the intubation was necessary, and whether all appropriate safety measures and methods to confirm placement were in place. If an endotracheal tube placed by EMS is not in the trachea, it is still possible that the EMS providers did everything correctly. Sometimes tubes are dislodged when moving the patient, sometimes the tube migrates, and sometimes inadequate sedation can allow the patients to dislodge it. But even in cases where a root cause cannot be identified, feedback should be given to the agency and the medic involved concerning the problem so that they can review the call themselves and determine what could be done to improve the outcome in the future. It is also important to instruct EMS agencies that even though they may be unable to document the circumstances of the call in real time, they should immediately complete their documentation as soon after the call as possible. This contemporaneous documentation is incredibly useful in the PI process, and in the possible defense of the malpractice action if one should be instituted.

As in most aspects of trauma performance improvement, the trauma program has little authority over EMS agencies. In our center, both myself and the associate trauma medical director work with EMS as operational medical directors. This allows us to gain insight into EMS operations and also provides a ready conduit for performance improvement inquiries and corrective action plans.

Transfer Hospitals

For level I and level II trauma centers, interactions with transferring hospitals can be a tremendous source of frustration. In general, hospitals that are not designated have decided that they do not want to provide optimal care for the injured patients. They may have outstanding doctors and nurses and support staff, but they do not have an organized response to critical injured patients in the vast majority of cases. Therefore, the workup can be disjointed, evaluation can be incomplete, and information provided can be erroneous. Also, nondesignated hospitals often do not know how trauma centers function. The last experience many emergency medicine physicians and surgeons at these hospitals had at a trauma center care was during their training. So they have been functioning, sometimes for decades, outside of the standard practice of designated trauma centers. I have often found that asking the centers to perform a state-of-the-art workup, or resuscitation is met with resistance and that "this is not necessary and not what we do here." Unfortunately, many of us give up at this point and just tell the referring hospital to get the patient to us as quickly as possible.

There are many ways to get solid closed-loop communication with transferring hospitals. The method that we use, and that many other hospitals use is a transfer center number for outside hospitals to use. The personnel manning that phone line will then ascertain that this is a request for transfer of a critical trauma patient and then will connect the emergency medicine physician working that day on the line, and in many hospitals the trauma surgeon on call will also be put on the line. There are many hospitals where the trauma surgeon is not included on this call and while that is acceptable, it can lead to delays and incorrect transfer of information, especially if the emergency medicine physician is extremely busy and is not able to take the time to call the trauma surgeon. We added the trauma surgeon for these calls in response to several PI events where the emergency room had 10 to 15 minutes more warning than the trauma team leading to suboptimal resuscitation in response to the patient's arrival.

The American College of Surgeons does require that the trauma center have a consistent method of communicating with their most frequent referring hospitals and provide them with follow-up information on the course of the patient they transferred. It is also important for site visitors if there were problems with the care provided at the referring hospital, that the trauma center PI program did make efforts to bring this problem to the referring hospital's attention and to try to work with them to ensure that it does not recur. There are many ways to do this. Our trauma program manager and PI coordinator have created a form that contains all necessary follow-up information that is transmitted back to the referring hospital on patient discharge.

Here are some of the common issues with referring hospitals:

- Inaccurate report of patient condition
- Missing records
- Missing X-rays
- Providing incorrect information to the family
- Forcing EMS to pass patient through their emergency department before transferring to trauma center
- If meeting a helicopter and using the hospital as a landing zone, telling EMS to bring patient into emergency department instead of allowing them to immediatley board the helicopter and begin transport.
- Inadequate resuscitation
- Poor vascular access
- Avoiding intubation when intubation is necessary
- Avoiding procedures when procedures are necessary

This is just an incomplete list and obviously trauma centers can be as guilty of these problems as referring community hospitals. However, most community hospitals (if not all) do not have a PI program that focuses on trauma. In fact, most do not have a mechanism to review trauma patients that pass through their emergency department who are transferred.

Vignette #5

We had a series of patients transferred from a community hospital approximately 35 miles away where care was significantly delayed in their emergency department. This hospital was located in the county where scene transport by helicopters of injured patients was less common than in other similar counties. One of the emergency department physicians is also the operational medical director for local rescue squads. This physician ordered the EMS agencies to avoid helicopter transport from the scene and instead had them bring the patient to the emergency department. I do not want to put any financial motives behind this, but in many cases, it was difficult to discern a reason why the patient should divert to the emergency department. We undertook a major effort to work with this hospital, the local EMS agencies, and the emergency department physicians in this hospital to try to optimize the situation. The hospital emergency department reasoning was that providing blood and/or procedures to these patients could be lifesaving. Endotracheal innovation was not really an issue since the aeromedical crews that work with our trauma center do an exceptional job with airway management. They were mostly referring to chest tube placement and the administration of blood products. We went back and audited all transfers from the emergency department and found that there were several instances where blood transfusion was begun, and actually these were very injured patients who had a much higher mortality rate. It was truly difficult to justify the time taken to move the patient the emergency department, get them through the initial phases, diagnose the need for a chest tube, place a chest tube, contact us for transfer, and then begin the transfer of the patient with the associated transport time and compare this to simply having the helicopter fly directly to us. We showed the hospital this data and explained that only in extremely rare situations would a delay in their emergency department benefit critically injured trauma patients. We also had to be mindful that even in our own studies, up to 60% of helicopter transports from this county and its adjoining county were deemed to be not medically necessary and did not meet the accepted national criteria for aeromedical transport of injured patients. So we want to walk a fine line between unnecessarily transporting patients by air and avoiding delays in the care of critically injured patients. In working with this emergency department, the aeromedical agencies, and local EMS we were able to determine a set of criteria where direct scene to trauma center transport would take place without delay. We also worked with this hospital to streamline their processes in the emergency department to ensure that critical patients spend as little time as possible there. We audited this for 6 months and found that delays from bypassing to their hospital were decreased, and there was a slight improvement in outcomes.

This is an example where having your trauma program involved with EMS in your region can be helpful. We would have never known the extent of this problem if we had not had contact with EMS and the aeromedical community. It is often difficult for site visitors to categorize what outreach is necessary to your regional referring hospitals. Really all that you need to show is that you are providing feedback of some sort. However, I think top trauma centers have their tendrils deep into the care of trauma patients and their surrounding regions. It is critical to build relationships with the key players in these counties which often include fire chiefs and EMS supervisors. It is also occasionally necessary to go above the emergency department in these referring hospitals and speak to their chief medical officers or administration directly especially if you feel that delays are worsening outcomes of your patients. We are in a situation where we are the only trauma center for 20,000 mi.^{2} so that these referring hospitals really do not have other choices for trauma care. We do realize how much more complex this is when there are multiple trauma centers that referring hospitals can choose from especially in urban areas. In those areas it is necessary for the trauma PI program to maintain close ties with referring hospitals and regional EMS management.

Chapter 12
Complex Opportunities for Improvement and Difficult Loop Closure

Physician Practice and Disagreement Among Specialists

Spine surgery is one of the more confusing areas of subspecialization among orthopedist and neurosurgeons. In almost every hospital, neurosurgery and orthopedics share spine call. Often, but not always, orthopedics is involved in more complex instrumentation of the spine, and neurosurgery is involved in more work with the discs and the spinal cord itself. However, these rules often do not apply, and the practices can overlap almost completely.

This overlap and frequent differences in philosophy between orthopedics and neurosurgery regarding spine care can be particularly vexing for the trauma program. I do want to make generalizations, but in general, one or the other of the specialties either tends to be more aggressive, or less aggressive than the other. This leads to difficulty in trying to come up with consistent ways to: image patients with suspected spine injuries, to create consistency in when they can be mobilized, determine timing for administration of thromboprophylaxis, and the timing of spinal fixation.

What follows is an interesting example of how a PI event could lead down a complex road that will eventually improve your program. We have, as most hospitals do, a robust process for identifying patients with healthcare-associated pressure ulcers. All patients are surveyed once a week, and the ICU has extensive procedures for changing skin contact for patients. We were notified by the ICU and the hospital about a pressure ulcer in one of our patients. It was somewhat surprising that the patient was not very injured and had burst fracture of the spine, some rib fractures, and an insignificant pelvic fracture. However, in drilling down on the case, we found that the patient was In bed, with spine precautions only being log rolled for 72 hours. After 72 hours, upright films were obtained and the patient's spine was cleared without any price. Therefore, this was a completely preventable pressure ulcer.

J. S. Young, *Trauma Center Performance Improvement*,
https://doi.org/10.1007/978-3-030-71048-4_12

In going through the patient care notes, we found that despite our team continually pressing to get the patient up, get the needed X-rays, and get clearance from the spine team, the spine team continued to delay and demand X-rays that we were unable to rapidly attain. Their initial recommendations were for an MRI of the spine, however due to the timing of the patient's admission, a full MRI schedule, and some relative contraindications, MRI for this patient was delayed and no other methods of clearance was attempted. Finally, the trauma director had to intervene and speak directly to the spine attending, telling them that MRI was just not going to happen and they had to figure out something else to do to get the patient mobilized. After another 24 hours of gnashing teeth, they relented and allowed us to upright films which still took 6 hours to obtain, but were normal and the patient was mobilized.

This incident prompted us to do a thorough reevaluation of our guidelines for spine injuries. We have tried many times in the past to gain some consensus, but those attempts involved having a liaison from the orthopedic team, and a liaison from the neurosurgery spine team following parallel paths, and then trying to reconcile the two guidelines. While we were able to get some very simple consensus, we were unable to get consensus concerning the indicated test for spine clearance, and when to start anticoagulation. We have had life-threatening thrombotic events appear in patients where DVT prophylaxis was delayed. For some time, we accepted the parallel pathways for the treatment and evaluation of spinal injuries, and every morning the trauma attending would ask which team was on for spine this month, knowing that we had to follow their guidelines. Sometimes the patient will be admitted on the 31st of the month under one team and then switch to the next team the next day.

We finally made a successful attempt in choosing one respected senior spine surgeon to spearhead the effort. We invited the surgeon to our PI meetings, helped gather whatever data he needed, and work closely with him to look at national guidelines and develop something that both sides could agree on. Though this did take some time, the gravitas that the surgeon had as the leading spine surgeon, the institution was able to overcome resistance from the opposing specialty group, and finally we were able to codify a set of guidelines that help to streamline care.

Nursing and Hospital Practice

Opportunities for improvement involving nursing practice can be extremely difficult and complex. The nursing practice structure usually leads up to the chief nursing officer and is usually entirely separate from the physician structure. Chief nursing officers of most institutions have great discretion in how they organize, how the nurses carry out their jobs, how they are disciplined and hired, and how they respond to care concerns. Below is an example of a complex nursing practice issue:

- Two trauma activations arrived in the surgical intensive care unit in the same hour. Both were critically ill and both require blood transfusions. Both also had anonymous trauma numbers which in our institution starts with a T, then the sex, and then a nine-digit medical record number. This system of anonymous naming was changed after this case.

- Blood was ordered for both patients from the blood bank. Patient 1's medical record number was TM9013465 and the second was TM9016466.When the blood arrived in the ICU through the pneumatic tube system, a patient care assistant picked up both containers of blood and brought them to the two ICU rooms which were two rooms apart. Including a variety of common errors, a full triple check was not performed on the blood, and in one room the blood administration was started. In the second room, a triple check was performed and was immediately realized that they did not have the correct blood products for their patient. They then rapidly notify the other room the transfusion was stopped and appropriate measures were taken. No harm came to the first patient.

Blood administration errors are extremely serious for the hospital, the patient, and regulatory agencies. In this case, the blood bank had done everything correctly, the blood indicated for the particular patient was properly crossmatched and was sent to the correct unit and was properly labeled. The error began to manifest once the blood arrived in the pneumatic tube system. There was no procedure detailing who would do the initial check on the blood and who would determine what patient the blood would be brought to. It was found that this was a fairly improvised system with few double checks and safety measures.

An important principle performance improvement arises from this case, which is to avoid blaming the nurse for a system that was poorly designed. This nurse was doing many tasks simultaneously and was dealing with the critically ill patient when she did not perform all the safety checks. There were several conditions that predisposed to error: first was the naming system by which only one digit was different between the patients, the next was that no safety checks or identity checks of any real death were done before the blood products were set on a table in a certain patient's room thus leading to bias on the part of the nurse that the correct blood products had been brought to the correct room. While it would be easy to blame the bedside nurse it, does not correct the system that may have led to many near misses that the trauma program was not made aware.

While there had been many near misses, this error prompted a changing in the naming system. This was also coincident with our electronic medical records upgrade which made it impossible to put medical record numbers in the patient's name. After looking at several other institutions, we decided on a list of all the countries in the world and rotated these in naming anonymous patients. Initially we have used to word names for colors that were recommended by our electronic medical record vendor. However it quickly became apparent that this was untenable in that even though the color may say canary yellow, on the residence list they just saw several patients whose last name was yellow which was very confusing and was right for error. Therefore, rotating country names was used and this is now been in place for several years with no significant errors or near misses reported.

Next was the process by which blood products are checked once they arrive in the ICU. Most blood products arrived by the pneumatic tube system and the system by which the initial contact was made at the tube station was solidified such that a nurse would do this initial check of the patient's name, medical record number, and room; initial the label; and then bring it to the room and at the doorway, not inside the room. A nurse inside the room would come to the door and perform the safety checks again at that point. This would again be the initial check, and then there will be the final safety check by the primary nurse before administration. Needless to say this was much more complicated and the actual process went through several iterations, but eventually it settled into a safe process for obtaining and administering blood in patients who needed urgently. We also looked at our massive transfusion protocol and attempted to make a determination of when we should switch from giving universal blood to type and crossed blood. We discussed this with the blood bank and created a guideline which was put in place.

We then audited blood transfusions in the ICU for 6 months and audited whether the process was working and found that the process was stable and no further near misses occurred. There were instances where the first safety check failed and the blood was bought to the wrong room; however, the second safety check at the gateway to the room caught all these issues.

Conflict with Hospital Quality Programs

An interesting problem that arises in many hospitals is the lack of integration between the hospital quality program and the trauma program. The American College of Surgeons does require that there be communication between the two programs but does not really specify like how this was done.

Hospital quality programs are constrained by the requirements of the joint commission. This includes definitions of sentinel events which the hospital must investigate and report to their quality committee. The search requirements do not exist for the trauma quality program of the American College of Surgeons and does require certain mandatory activities such as reviews of deaths among other filters. Some hospitals have a very long time for closure of cases within their hospital quality program. The most common problem is when the trauma program rapidly adjudicates the case but it is required to send that case to the hospital quality program for further activity. On many site visits, I have seen cases that were rapidly analyzed by the trauma program that then sat with the hospital quality program for half a year. Obviously, the trauma program has only so much influence over this timeline. It is important for the site reviewer to be mindful of the restrictions under which the quality program of the trauma center works. However, the site visit is the one opportunity where external judges can strongly indicate to the hospital that they must provide loop closure on cases referred for the trauma program as quickly as possible in the cases that cannot take months and months to close. We often have to work with whatever the trauma program came up with regarding the closure. However for issues such as nursing practice as I detailed above, respiratory therapy practice, blood draws, ITE, and other issues, the trauma program does not have the authority to make a change in these areas, and thus the hospital quality program is the only entity able to implement certain corrective action plans in these areas. This can be an extremely vexing problem for high-performing trauma PI programs, and the only solution is to work closely with your hospital quality program. It is imperative that the lead players in trauma program PI sit on committees and have significant input in the hospital quality structure. It is also important that the output of the trauma program PI system be integrated into the hospital system for the trauma program protection and for loop closure for the hospital. It is not a good idea for the two programs to be siloed and operate completely independently in that both programs can learn from each other and both programs need the other program to implement change.

Financial Limitations

Performance improvement opportunities that involve finances can be the most vexing of all. All hospitals have to worry about their margin and their cost and revenue. It is a balance between obtaining all the equipment, personnel, and capabilities that any clinician may want, and the realization that if they do not generate a margin they cannot stay in business.

Issues that arise from financial considerations include adequate personnel, adequate equipment, sufficient radiology capability, sufficient ICU space, optimal equipment, among many others. The key with regard to these PI opportunities is effort. Your site visitors know that you cannot possibly mandate to the hospital that they spend considerable sums of money for trauma patients that may only affect those patients. The site visitors want to see you demonstrate that there is a need for additional resources that you vigorously presented this to administration and that there is documentation from the administration as to why they did not grant the finances for these resources. Although effort counts in most instances if the site visit team determines that due to multiple denials for resources you are affecting the outcome of patients, then the team may assign one of the most damning deficiencies which is inadequate commitment to trauma care. Sometimes trauma programs will use a site visit as leverage to obtain resources that they feel are essential to providing optimal care.

FTEs

Having adequate personnel to properly care for trauma patients is a problem that all centers face. There are some states that mandate nurse staffing ratios through legislation or through nursing unions, but the majority of states do not have such regulations. The American College of Surgeons requires that the nurse to patient ratio in the intensive care unit be no more than 1:2, but beyond that there are not criterion related to this topic. The site visit team can, through the examination of cases, determine that nursing, respiratory therapy, or other clinicians staffing contributed to multiple events. Should that be the case, program must demonstrate considerable effort in trying to present their case that additional staffing is needed to provide optimal care. One problem many places face is having enough personnel to handle every reasonable situation. For instance, in academic centers, many advanced practice practitioners do not work in the hospital during night shifts or throughout the weekends. This may lead to standards of care where during the week and experienced nurse practitioners and physician assistants provide acute care and ICU treatment while on nights and weekends cross covering lower-level residents do this. There is no hard and fast rule of this, however, if case analysis demonstrates significant opportunities for improvement based on two standards of care, then it is incumbent upon the program to ensure that they present this vigorously to the hospital and ask for additional resources. However, few hospitals have unlimited funds to staff their wards 24 – seven – 365 with advanced practice practitioners at ratios which the trauma program may demand.

In most cases, the solution to this sort of financial gap is for the program to institute guidelines and procedures that can limit the variability of the care provided on nights and weekends. If you see that staffing in the hospital drops drastically after the sun goes down, then you may very well be asked what you are doing about it. This is especially true should this have adversely affected a patient's outcome. In these PI cases, the creation of consensus guidelines for response and treatment to common nighttime and weekend clinical changes are usually necessary along with continued monitoring that these changes in patient condition are being responded to appropriately. It is not sufficient for a program to throw their hands up in the air and say we asked for more staff and they denied. This happens in every program and the best programs deal with this adversity by training, education, and trying to decrease variability at all hours of day and night.

But if you do feel there is a possibility that you can obtain more FTEs, the program should do several things to improve their argument. The first is to show that this increased staff could benefit hospital metrics. For instance, additional ICU, or acute care floor staff, or advanced practice practitioners can decrease length of stay, complications, and improve metrics used for benchmarking by national organizations. Of course, if the addition of these FTEs do none of these things, then the program should be prepared that these spots may be taken away. However, it is rare that a hospital will remove an FTE after creating the position, which is the reason why they are usually extremely careful about increasing their number of staff. Another strategy is to appeal to the standard of care. If your PI case demonstrates that care fell below the standard due to staffing and that there was an adverse patient outcome, this of course can be a strong argument. However, it needs to be shown that this is not a "one-off" situation, where it is unlikely that the same variables will be present commonly in the future. A way to enhance this argument is to look at the exact factors that contributed to the patient's poor outcome and cogently argue that there are a few other interventions that could be done to decrease these risks other than adding personnel. It is also important that the program be cognizant of the fact that you may require additional personnel during your busy trauma months, whereas these personnel would not be used at all during your slower months. The best and most effective arguments demonstrate that additional personnel will improve metrics, improve hospital margin, and will be applied consistently throughout the year. An even stronger argument could be made that these personnel, such as advanced practice practitioners, could be used across services thus being force multipliers.

Equipment

Another common and difficult problem is adequate equipment. This can range from very expensive MRIs, spine and fracture tables, orthopedic implants, two ultrasound machines in the ICU and the emergency department, or PPE. As I stated above the most effective arguments for disbursement of money to buy additional equipment revolve around improving patient outcomes, improving hospital metrics, and generalizability. If one orthopedic surgeon wants one very expensive implant, and no other orthopedic surgeon feels the same, then the trauma program may not want to support obtaining this equipment unless it can be clearly demonstrated that it will raise the level of care provided to the patient. In our own facility, we were able to obtain a major outlay of funds to obtain multiple trauma carts. These carts are used in our resuscitation bays and contain all the equipment we may need to place chest tubes, and the bleeding wounds, place arterial and central lines, etc. The cart method also allowed us to create a surplus of 8 to 10 carts which could be used for multiple casualty incidents. Essentially these carts could be brought to any bed in the hospital and converted into a reasonably equipped trauma bay. In addition, the carts are sealed and whenever a seal is broken they are brought to central supply and completely checked and resupplied. This ensures that the equipment that is supposed to be on the cart is always on the part if the seal is intact. We were able to convince our institution by arguing that having the court system would free up time for the emergency department staff, that it was the corrective action plan of multiple events where equipment is not available, and that it provides an excellent answer to the question of how we would obtain equipment to convert a regular bed into a trauma bed should we have multiple casualties.

A delicate issue is having adequate trauma program staff. The American College of Surgeons has someone vacillated on the number of registrars needed for each program. It has ranged from 500 to 750 cases per registrar, but I have seen few centers that have one registrar for every 500 patients. However, most programs will have a registrar for every 750 patients. Again if you need more registry help it is important to frame the request on the need to meet regulatory requirements, the ability to submit to TQIP for national benchmarking, delays in PI activities due to lack of registry support, and the inability to supply data to the hospital and other departments because the limited number of registrars are spending all their time abstracting charts.

Another personnel issue within trauma programs is adding a PI coordinator. I can say without hesitation that programs that see over 1500 cases a year that have a dedicated PI coordinator appeared, at least to me, to have more efficient and effective PI programs. There really is no substitute for having an experienced nurse whose sole job is to identify, analyze, present, and fixed PI problems. Often the trauma program manager has more than enough on their plate such that PI activities are merely one of the many activities that are part of their job. Registrars do not usually carry out analysis and corrective action plan creation. The trauma medical director in smaller programs may need to keep up their clinical practice for financial survival and cannot dedicate time every day to the basics of PI. Thus, it is obvious that having a separate PI coordinator can enhance performance. The American College of Surgeons does not require this because every program has different needs, but my own recommendation is that if it is all possible, the program should have a PI coordinator. Obtaining a PI coordinator from the hospital can often be difficult. If you have not been verified in the site visit due to PI activities, then that can be used as leverage to obtain this position. It can be hard if you have had superior performance in your site visits to justify it. One argument that is becoming more common is that most major trauma programs do have a PI coordinator position, and this can be used to try to influence administration to keep up with what other centers are doing.

In summary, getting the hospital to spend money on the trauma program can be very frustrating. The program cannot effectively use the excuse of lack of personnel in a multitude of PI cases unless it wishes to demonstrate that the hospital simply does not have the commitment to being a trauma center. I have outlined some strategies that can be used to try to influence a hospital to fund additional personnel, equipment, or resources to enhance the care of injured patients.

The Interdepartmental Conflict

Interdepartmental conflicts can be very difficult to resolve. I have already discussed the issues with spine care where orthopedics and neurosurgery are essentially switching off on caring for roughly the same population of patients with sometimes very different philosophies toward diagnosis and treatment. It can be very difficult for the trauma medical director get in the middle of this, and as I said previously the best strategy is to use national guidelines and evidence and consensus building to try to influence cooperation.

Perhaps the greatest source of conflict for most trauma programs is with the emergency department. The trauma program spends a significant amount of its effort in the emergency department, and subpar performance by the emergency department and setback of patients care tremendously.

One of the more common areas of conflict is the activation process. Many emergency physicians do not like the idea of rigid guidelines for calling the trauma team. Emergency department nurses and staff often feel that the trauma team can be disruptive, they can cause crowding, and that they setback care for other patients. My hope would be that the organization of your trauma response is such that these criticisms are not true, and it is incumbent upon trauma program leadership to ensure that the trauma response is not unduly burdening emergency department. The American College of Surgeons can help with this problem by mandating a set of criteria that must lead to trauma team activation. It is not possible for a center that wishes to be verified by the ACS to leave out any of these criteria. The problem usually arises with second-tier criteria. These can include mechanism, age, conditions such as pregnancy or age, specific injuries, or specific combinations of injuries and conditions. Hospitals will often have one set of trauma team activation criteria, but this can lead to burnout on the part of the trauma team when they are responding within 15 minutes for patients that clearly do not warrant that type of response.

Lack of Hospital or Clinician Commitment

I have touched on this in other chapters, but clinician or hospital ambivalence toward trauma care is very likely the most difficult problem to correct. Hospital administrators, owners, and CEOs have a variety of problems that they need to deal with. These include market share, profitability, costs, revenue, etc. If the hospital leadership is determined that caring for injured patients at a high level is not in the best interest of their facility, there is going to be very little that the trauma program can do to influence this. They can develop arguments regarding competition and devotion to the citizens in their community to try to move leadership toward greater engagement in trauma care; however, it is likely that the leadership authority heard these arguments. What is more important is how the trauma program deals with this issue.

Regarding clinician commitment, lack of commitment is often demonstrated by unwillingness to take call, unwillingness to respond trauma activations, lackluster involvement in the care of the patients from resuscitation to discharge, irrational opposition to trauma program initiatives, resistance to the development of guidelines to try to streamline care, among many others. I have seen clinicians in trauma centers that exhibit one or more of these problems. A simple solution when available is to remove the clinician from the trauma however, as I have seen if the clinician is the department chair, a division Chief, or a prominent surgeon within the community it can be very difficult especially for a junior trauma director to take this step. However, it must be realized that when the site visit team comes in and sees a variety of adverse events attributed to a single clinician, and also sees a complete lack of attempts at corrective action, then this raises significant concerns. It would be easy for me to say that any clinician can be removed from trauma care, but I know that this can also be extremely difficult and political in many departments in hospitals. As I said previously the key here is effort. Most experienced reviewers are well aware of the political considerations in medical care. What they do not want to see is "we can't do anything about this" and the program tolerating dangerous or lazy care. They will want to see documented conversations with the clinician, and if that fails escalation up through the hospital structure to try to develop a remedy. I would say that in my experience truly substandard clinician performance can be dealt with. Either the amount of call of this person takes is greatly reduced, or the clinician becomes convinced that is simply more trouble and is worth to continue to be part of the trauma program.

I am not stating that the solution to this problem is always separation from the program, but that always has to be on the table. Site visit teams will grow very concerned if they see consistent documentation of problems, attempted interventions, and then continued evidence of problems with a single clinician. The program should extensively document the analysis of any case with an adverse event, document the conversations with the clinician, document how follow-up was done, and demonstrate that noncompliance was not tolerated and that the problem was escalated through the hospital hierarchy. There will always be weak players in any group of clinicians taking care for injured patients. The best thing that a trauma program can do is design a consistent, low variability trauma care delivery system that decreases the amount of mayhem that a single clinician can introduce. If you have a clinician that is simply not doing their job, demonstrating that you have made the effort not only to address the individual clinician, but to address the care process in such a way to make individual clinician performance less critical to optimal outcomes.

Regarding lack of hospital commitment, as I said previously that trauma program must undertake efforts to educate hospital leadership as to the necessity and the benefits of being a verified trauma center. Lack of hospital commitment can be demonstrated in many ways including refusing to hire adequate personnel, refusing to obtain necessary equipment, refusing to pay stipends to subspecialty physicians that are critical to designation, placing undue burdens on trauma program physicians, or consistently focusing on financial outcomes instead of clinical outcomes. Financial outcomes are important but they cannot override the majority of clinical concerns. When a trauma program faces a hospital that intrinsically or through the introduction of a new management team decides that being a trauma center is not for them, and after they have expended effort to attend to educate leadership as to what is necessary to provide optimal trauma care, they may have to face the fact that they should not be a trauma center. On several visits I have said "not every hospital needs to be a trauma center." I say this when it is clear that the facility simply does not have the commitment as exemplified by many of the factors I described above, the care is substandard, and there really is no plan to correct their deficiencies. I have visited facilities that have terminated their efforts to become trauma centers, or to continue to be a trauma center after review. But it is very likely that the review plays little role in this and that the facility on the program realize that they were on thin ice and they were not providing the right level of care to their citizens. It is not shameful to be a nondesignated hospital, there are far more undesignated hospitals in this country than designated trauma centers. If your hospital determines that it no longer wishes to be designated as a trauma center, should the trauma program staff continue to work there, then they should continue to try to influence the emergency department and other clinicians to properly resuscitate patients and transfer them expeditiously. In my work with my own state, the worst combination of events is a hospital that is unwilling to put forth the effort and resources to become designated, and also has an inflated view of their own ability to take care of trauma patients. This leads to inadequate care, late transfer, and complications and death and should not be tolerated from a system perspective. Though many states do not provide remedy for hospitals that decide to act this way, again significant efforts should be made by those individuals that participate in the administration of the trauma program for the state to protect the citizens being served by these hospitals.

Chapter 13
Inspection of PI Process by Reviewers

We now begin to address the meat of the matter which is how to prepare your trauma center for a site visit by either a state or national entity. As I said previously, I have extensive experience in site visiting trauma centers both for state agencies and for the American College of Surgeons as well as having passed, without any deficiencies, several ACS level-I site visits.

I invite readers to also look at my other publication *Trauma Centers: A Quick Guide* [1] also published by Springer Verlag since I devote a significant part of the latter half of that book to site visit preparation. I will go over some of those issues again here, but I do invite you to read both what I write here and what I wrote in the other book.

Chart and Document Setup

Nothing is quite as annoying to a site visitor or regulator than haphazard and poorly put together documents and medical records. You can easily control the flow of review from a site visitor or inspector by properly setting up your documents and charts in such a way that they tell the story that you want to tell in the way that you want to tell it. Allowing inspectors or site reviewers to merely forage through medical records and documents without any direction is a recipe for disaster. First of all it will anger the inspectors and site reviewers that you have not taken sufficient time to put your records together. There are more-than-enough resources out there (including my own previous publication) and documents provided by state entities and the American College of Surgeons that outline how documents and records should be put together. I have been on more visits than I can count where despite being clearly told what records needed to be reproduced and gathered for the inspection, the programs completely ignored this guidance, printed out every single page of the medical record (often thousands of pages), and simply putting a Post-it note

© The Author(s), under exclusive license to Springer Nature Switzerland AG 2021
J. S. Young, *Trauma Center Performance Improvement*,
https://doi.org/10.1007/978-3-030-71048-4_13

on them and stacking them up. Even the most experienced site reviewer in the world cannot easily go through an electronic medical record that is simply printed in its entirety without any attempt at organization in any reasonable period of time.

I think it is incredibly important that the trauma program go through their medical records and documents as if they were a reviewer and were seeing them for the first time. For each of our site visits whether done by the state or the college, I looked through every single record that we are going to present to the reviewers and go through each page to see that it is accurate, is reflecting our efforts, and if there were significant problems that we could not address includes our meeting minutes, discussions, and other materials that exemplify the effort that we put forth to try to correct problems. As I said previously, you should never try to hide problematic issues since they will almost certainly be found. Reviewers can be very lenient with a program that is honest about their problems and their attempts to correct them. But a dishonest program will not be viewed positively. The best strategy is to honestly present the truth. Beyond that the absolute best strategy is to have an extremely effective PI program where you can effectively address most of the opportunities for improvement that present themselves. Nobody expects every OFI to be addressed with perfect loop closure and documentation, but it is expected that opportunities stemming from adverse events, death, applications, or significant impediments to optimal care be reviewed extensively and that significant efforts are put in to corrective action.

Remember if you do not write down you did not do it. I have been on several visits where a sparse PI record for a significant case is brought to the attention of the trauma program staff and then they all look at each other and state "oh that's Bill" and then proceed to regale us with 20 minutes of the case history, PI efforts, and loop closure. While this is certainly okay, we would certainly prefer that the majority of the effort be documented and that we can fill in some blanks through conversation with trauma program staff rather and have nothing documented in here about the entire process verbally. If you have significant issues related to the PI of a case, it should be in the PI record that you present to the site reviewer. You do not need to re-create parts of the chart in the PI record but you do need to document critical factors in PI review.

We set up our folders for site visits in the following manner. I am not saying this is the only way to do it, but our process is the product of the hundreds of site visits that I have done.

First for deaths, there needs to be a folder for each event. The death should be categorized according to the categories that the ACS provides. They should not all be lumped together. Unanticipated deaths with opportunities for improvement should be first and anticipated deaths without opportunity for improvement should be in the last folder. All of the church in a certain category should be placed in a separate box, or if doing electronically in a separate folder. As an aside I would be extremely careful about doing the entire documentation for a visit electronically. Many things can go wrong, computer access can be lost, computers can go down, files can be misplaced, etc. Therefore, I would recommend that paper should be used for PI charts and the documents can be printed out from electronic records.

The categories of the ACS, and other state agencies, require may differ but in general I leave all the charts pertaining to a single category should be in one box.

The folders that contain performance improvement activities should be placed in the front and should be marked appropriately. Each box should also have a list of the charts that are within the box along with category, age, sex, name, medical record number, injury severity score, and a column for whether PI activities to place on the chart.

On the front of each folder we affix a sticker that contains only information that the reviewer would need to decide whether to examine the chart. It includes information I stated above as well as the category that the church fits into. We have a separate process from other centers with regard to multiple related events that are aggregated into center-wide PI projects. For instance, if you are looking at availability of CT scanning on weekends (which should not be a problem in level I but I am only using as an example) and this affected for example 25 charts in the site visit period, it can be disorganized for the same corrective action plan to be copied and reprinted into 25 separate charts. What we do is for aggregated opportunities for improvement in the individual chart we indicate that the PI analysis corrective action and loop closure are included in the project folder, and then the project folder lists the process by which we corrected the opportunity and the medical record numbers or chart designations of the patients who were affected by the opportunity for improvement. We have found this not only allows us to show off major projects demonstrating the capabilities of the PI program to handle tough issues, but is also more efficient for the site reviewers. Currently, the ACS is piloting a system by which the charts that will be reviewed or decided on beforehand and it is important that the spreadsheet that you provide to the ACS speak very accurate and easy to interpret.

We use manila folders that have binder clips on both sides of the folder internally. On the left side of the folder, we place the PI records including the fascia from the registry, the trauma PI intake sheet, all the documentation concerning identification of OFIs, discussion at meetings, discussions with clinicians, and discussions with administrative personnel. We then ensure that the corrective action plan is clearly marked and accurately described, and then place a separate category for loop closure and provide the documents supporting loop closure on that sheet. On the right side of the chart, we place the records required by the designating agency whatever they may be. The American College of Surgeons includes the EMS run sheet, the trauma flowsheet, the trauma history and physical, any operations done in the first 24 hours, and the discharge summary. This is only a minimum document, but it allows the reviewer to survey the case and determine what other documents or results they need to examine.

Content of Documents

There are many ways to set up the documents. I can just give you my opinion for my extensive experience. Try as best you can and do not to provide a spreadsheet with 20 different patient entries in it from a PI meeting where only one of those entries is relevant to that chart. Using PDFs and other methods you can extract only the relevant part of the minutes from the meeting and include that rather than forcing the reviewer to review large spreadsheets to find what they need. You can also simply print out records and highlight key data

Ensure that you provide all of the benchmarking and metrics necessary for the reviewers to properly examine the chart. This includes at the very least the injury severity score, but we prefer to put the probability of survival on the chart as well. You should also include length of stay, ICU length of stay, adverse events, and discharge destination on a single document that is easy for the reviewer to look at.

There is no reason why you cannot highlight portions of the medical record that you have copied and placed in the site visit chart in order to bring them to the reviewer's attention. In fact, I would recommend that rather than forcing the reviewer to look through dozens and dozens of pages of records to find what they need. As I said previously, the only way that you will set up a chart as efficiently as possible is for you to look at the chart with a clean slate and attempt to follow the story of the patient's care and the performance improvement going from front to back. When you do this, you will really easily identify problems with the way that the record to set up that inhibit your ability to truly understand what is going on.

It is an extremely common occurrence during site visits for a program to have done an exemplary job with performance improvement but give the site reviewer the impression that they did a shoddy job. This occurs because the documentation is poor, they are not readily available to provide fill-in-the-blank information for the reviewers should they need it, there are errors in the chart such as having the wrong record in the wrong place, and more importantly as I stated before having one or two sentences to describe an extremely complex discussion and creation of a corrective action plan and expecting that the personnel present at the review will fill in the remaining large amount of material. You do not need to write everything down in the records of course but you do need to write enough to make sure that the reviewer does not have the impression that you are improvising. It does concern reviewers when there is little written in the chart that they are presented with and yet the trauma program staff can pontificate for minutes on minutes about the case. Your advice to the program should be that if significant performance improvement activities only exist by passing the information verbally from person to person that it is easy for that information to get lost and it demonstrates a suboptimal process for institutional and program memory.

So what do you need to put in the documents concerning your PI activities? As I said previously, you need the reviewer to be able to follow the patient's story from start to finish. In many jurisdictions, it was very difficult to obtain EMS documentation. We understand this and know that it can be difficult, but the hospital needs to spend some effort to obtain these materials. First, the patient's original condition when found by first responders is important. Second, the time course of the EMS treatment can be important. If there were undue delays or long transport times, or if unneeded procedures were done which delay the arrival of the patient the trauma center and allowed further degradation their condition, this is important part of the

PI process since the EMS agencies should be considered to be part of the trauma team and thus part of the trauma PI process.

Many EMS records contain a great deal of extraneous information but at the very least you want the patient's primary survey when they were first encountered, to be able to follow the time course of their vital signs during treatment and transport, and to look at the success of procedures that were performed en route. If the procedure is performed that went poorly, it is important that the trauma program to review the documentation to ascertain whether proper procedures were in place. One of the more common PI interactions with EMS is over failed intubation. If there is a field intubation, it is important for the program to look at how many attempts were made, whether placement was confirmed by an appropriate method, and whether there was adequate monitoring after the intubation to ensure that the two did not become dislodged, or that some other serious problem was impacting ventilation and oxygenation. While some site reviewer is like to have the source material immediately available, I have visited several trauma centers that merely summarized all of these points I stated above in prose form under EMS section of the PI records. I feel this is a very useful way of doing this in that it saves the reviewer time, and also saves the program time when they want to go back and evaluate EMS activities.

The second part of the documentation of the PI case is the trauma flowsheet from the emergency department. Once electronic medical records became ubiquitous throughout the country, there was great difficulty in obtaining a usable trauma flowsheet for PI activities and review. All trauma flowsheets were usually 1 to 3 pages of handwritten entries that flowed through the initial interaction with the patient, primary survey, vital signs, fluids, blood administration, procedures, who was present in the trauma bay and what time they arrived, and then the time when the patient left the trauma bay for either admission, the operating room, interventional procedures, etc.

There were certainly times when centers were in a transition period between paper flowsheet and electronic ones where a lot of material was lost. Most electronic medical record vendors, such as Epic, create extremely large documents when attempting to print what was in the computer system onto paper. These paper outputs can be very jumbled, contain an unbelievable amount of unused information, and can make it difficult to identify individual important source of information. If this is the case in your institution, you need to expend the effort to go through the printed trauma flowsheet from the electronic medical record and highlight and/or pull out the information that you know that the reviewers will need. Once again, I have to reiterate this in the strongest terms you should not force your reviewers to search for information. Any trauma program with any amount of experience should be well aware of what is necessary in the PI review and should not simply place a large number of printed sheets from the medical record in the PI review without any sifting, filtering, or highlighting. To the reviewer this shows a very cursory process of not only examining records but of collating and creating permanent PI records for later review and analysis.

In the ED, the registry needs the patient's initial condition on arrival, whether the trauma surgeon was present for a highest-level activation, consultant service arrival, data from the primary survey and initial vital signs, whether additional intravenous lines were placed and what the status were of the lines that may have been placed by EMS, if the patient requires intubation: what drugs were used, the time that it was done, and the method of checking placement. Programs should realize that the ED trauma flowsheet contains documentation of 60 to 70% of the actions by which a case will be judged. Certainly there are cases where the majority of the PI opportunity occurs after leaving the emergency department, but in many centers it is what goes on in the emergency department upon the arrival of the patient that reflects the quality of care of the trauma centers.

Following the ED flowsheet, you should print out the materials of the American College of Surgeons provides in their previsit instructions. I may miss some of this, but I believe it is EMS records, trauma flowsheet, trauma history and physical, discharge summary, and operative notes and procedures as well as the record created by the PI program. While many of us do not look at daily progress notes or the source data from radiology, some of us do and obviously you should have those available through either an electronic radiology record reviewing system, and access to the full EMR through workstations in the room where the reviewers are working. The history and physical is important to understand what the trauma services, or specialty services, initial impression of the patient was, and what their initial plan of attack was. If the patient is persistently hypotensive as evidenced by the flowsheet, and this is not mentioned in the history and physical, then obviously this is a problem. If the patient has severely abnormal lab values or study results, this must be reflected in the history and physical or through a note if the data becomes available after the history and physical has been created. Since in most institutions with training programs the attendings are required to cosign all resident and advanced practice practitioners notes at some point, just having a cosign does not indicate that the attending was present throughout the resuscitation nor that they even read the note. So if it is a complex dynamic situation requiring a great deal of advanced decision-making and this leads to an adverse outcome, it is important that the attending physician leave at least some small note of the thought processes. Even though most trauma program PI activities try to be conducted within a reasonable amount of time from the patient's admission, some cases, especially after long patient's days, may not come up for review for months. It is highly unlikely that the attending physician remember sufficient details about the case to be helpful to the PI investigation 3 to 4 months after the patient was admitted. I am well aware that attending physicians do not create a lot of notes in this modern age, but the trauma director should impress upon them the need to do this in those cases where there decision-making may be called into question, or where there are competing data leading to complex decisions. Subspecialty attendings (neurosurgery, orthopedics) rarely personally document in the chart. The trauma program should reiterate to them that if they make controversial decisions (such as not operating on a young patient with a large subdural), there needs to be adequate documentation from the attending or at least from a senior resident with affirmative documentation that they spoke directly to the attending about the decision.

There are many other pieces of information that can be placed in the PI record. But my personal opinion is I want to see operative notes from the first 24 hours and procedure notes from this time period as well. By looking at the anesthesia record, reviewers can often ascertain what time the patient arrived in the operating room and what time they left. It will also give them information about the amount of blood products patient received, and what their course was during operation. Since PI activities revolve around adverse events and adverse outcomes, there should be good documentation of how procedures were performed since complications from procedures are not infrequent.

Clearly the discharge summary is important in order for the reviewer, and the PI program, to understand how long the patient spent in the hospital, what procedures were done, what complications arose, and what their condition was upon discharge. If there were adverse events and rapid changes in patient's condition, the notations from the time period around those issues (such as rapid response team activation) be included in the PI record to better explain what role the care team may have had in causing or at least not preventing a major complication.

The PI record itself is by far the most important part of the documents that you present to reviewers. In addition, the PI record itself is incredibly important to the program since they can use this to go back and review previous cases and significant complications and look at the discussions and plans of action. Probably no two programs have the exact same format for their PI record. Many registry vendors have excellent forms that the registry can fill-in for consolidated document for review. At the very least, the PI document should contain much of the initial data I described above, but this is usually included since the required registry fields usually cover these areas, as well as the time course and reasons for review.

There is a wide range in the aggressiveness of PI programs and what they focus on. At the very least every death must be thoroughly evaluated as well as sentinel events and major complications, but some programs only do these things in some programs that are very busy looking at an extremely large number of opportunities that bear little on the outcome of the patient. This tends to tie up the PI program and prevent them from carrying out all the phases of PI activities. The reviewers can provide advice to the program as to what an experience trauma director views as critical opportunities for improvement and what others could be delegated to other entities within the hospital or simply are not appropriate for a full PI review.

Beyond the data extracted from the registry the PI record should indicate who did the initial review, what was the opinion of the original reviewer, what the recommendations were, and who they refer the case to. Many programs do this differently if the trauma program manager or trauma PI coordinator is given the independence to determine which cases go for further review and which may be closed. As an example, patient arrives with a gunshot wound to the head with cerebral matter displayed who dies rapidly in the emergency department can often be closed at the first-level review in many programs. In some programs, the decision is made by the initial reviewers, and then it is simply double-checked with the physician supervising the PI program. All of this should be documented. What I did for a long time was instead of looking at the deaths that had opportunities for improvement, I looked at five or six deaths that were closed by the program. While I in the vast majority cases felt few surprises, looking at deaths that the program determines to require no PI effort can be a good indication of the diligence of the program.

If the case goes to second, third, or fourth levels of review, the activities in each of these levels of review should be thoroughly documented and included in the records provided to the reviewers. For instance, if the trauma medical director adds their review to that of the trauma program manager, then there should be more than just a few scribbled words from the medical director in the record. It does not need to be voluminous but it does need to indicate some reasoning if, for instance, the medical director decides that they should be close while the program manager felt that there was an opportunity and vice versa. The medical director felt the case required for the review when the program manager felt the case to be closed. Getting insight into the reasoning and interactions within the trauma PI program really is important for reviewers to understand how the program functions and at what level.

The college requires that all deaths be reviewed by your multidisciplinary PI committee in some way. For anticipated deaths without opportunity for improvement, this can simply be done with the slide indicating some patient demographics, the mechanism of injury, the time course, and the disposition. Of course, programs should be insightful and aggressive toward review the deaths, but reviewing deaths that had no significant opportunities in patients with fatal injuries at several levels is simply a waste of time and effort. In most centers, the next level above the trauma program manager and trauma medical director is the multidisciplinary PI committee; however, some institutions, such as ours, inserted a committee between the PI committee and individual review. Many programs call this an "divisional PI meeting," or this step can be represented by morbidity and mortality discussions in various departments. In this meeting, cases are usually triaged, and the findings of initial review be discussed. These meetings can be very useful in busy programs where waiting for the monthly multidisciplinary committee often can delay loop closure. Truly all that is required at the multidisciplinary PI committee is that there is a review of major PI activities. The multidisciplinary committee's purpose is to allow all liaisons and various departments involved in injured patient care, to be brought together to discuss a case, as well as the corrective action plan. But there is nothing that prevents the program from doing intense analysis, discussion, and corrective action planning without the input of this committee. The multidisciplinary PI committee really needs to be the final stop for any cases can be closed and for displaying loop closure.

If you do have a committee between the key individuals and the multidisciplinary committee, the minutes from these meetings should not be extensive but should document the opportunities, their analysis, and recommendations. A very useful component of this intermediate committee is that it can take the time to review whatever tool the program uses to keep track of all of PI activities. In our program, several Excel spreadsheets are used to document all the stages of a review and cases are categorized as to whether they are close, open with corrective action plans in place, corrective action plans pending, or cases that have not yet had sufficient review. It can be difficult, especially in a busy program, to do this at the multidisciplinary meeting, since it requires a great deal of time, whereas a small committee meeting weekly can do the tactical assessment of where cases stand, and prioritize those cases that are still waiting in the queue.

Minutes from the multidisciplinary meeting must include at least a synopsis of the discussion at that meeting. If there is conflict between the recommendations made prior to the meeting and the output of the meeting, then obviously it is very important that the reasoning is documented. I am well aware that some states do not protect performance improvement materials; thus, programs in the states are very wary to put information in the meeting minutes that could be used in a court of law. However, the program must demonstrate their PI process. There are many ways of doing this and in the past several years I have found that most states that have this issue have figured out workarounds to be able to demonstrate analysis and loop closure to the site visit teams.

When providing information from the multidisciplinary meeting, please do not merely print out the entire record from that meeting and place it in the individual PI folder when that record only contains 10 or 20 words related to that case. If the documentation resides on a sheet that also contains documentation in many other cases, you do not need to pull that information out on a separate document; however, you should merely provide that page from the records of the PI meeting with the case of concern highlighted so that the reviewer does not need to go hunting. I have been in visits where critical information concerning the PI process was present in minutes printed out and placed individual PI records that were 10 or even 15 pages long and could not be found by the reviewer. Experienced reviewers will go to the program personnel and asked them to find it; however, you also would be taking the chance that inexperience reviews may conclude that no discussion occurred or that it was not documented. I cannot reiterate enough that before the site visit you must go through the charts you are presenting to the reviewers and ensure that all the information required for that reviewer to determine the quality of the PI process are easy to read and do not require effort to find.

To make things even easier for the reviewers, you can categorize cases that fall under the same corrective action plan in a single folder with documentation of the plan as well as the plan for auditing and loop closure. The individual PI record still needs to exist; however, you can place in each of those records a placeholder saying that the issue that was found related to, for example, appropriate trauma attending response the highest-level activations, and if this occurs in several cases and you undertook a global effort to improve this, you can merely say in the individual record that the corrective action plan – auditing – loop closure are included in a "PI project" folder that will be provided to the reviewer. We have done this on all of our reviews and it has been well received.

Finally ensure that the document that is available to the reviewers is properly collated, tabbed, and secured. There is nothing worse for a program that when a folder gets knocked off the table that all the pages scattered throughout the room or the review is occurring. If you went through this chart before the reviewers arrived, you would realize that materials need to be secured either with a binder clip or through some other attachment to the folder itself and that it needs to be placed in order that is easy for the reviewer to use. Again I recommend separating the PI records from the patient chart within that folder placing one on one side and one on the other so that it is not mixed in. This decreases the possibility of the reviewer missing important information. Also remember that while you may assume that the reviewer will ask for help if they cannot find something, sometimes reviews under time pressure, especially in combined adult pediatric reviews, and the reviewer may just conclude that something does not exist if they do not find it in the folder.

Supplemental Material

There are a variety of useful supplementary materials and can be available to the site reviewers. These include large posters that document guideline creation and major PI activities. These can be placed on the wall of the review room or on easels. First this provides an easy to read and access description of something the program is proud of, and allows the program personnel to have a one-on-one discussion with the reviewer about the opportunity and its correction. While it is required in another section, any program-wide or hospital-wide guidelines, policies, and procedures that are the output from a PI review should all be collated and provided to the reviewers. Every hospital should have a guideline manual for people coming onto the trauma service and for trauma practitioners to use on a daily basis and they should be available. The manual can be online, as ours is, and does not need to be printed out but signage for the reviewers should clearly indicate how they can access it. Reviewers will also want to know how often the protocols are reviewed, edited, and adapted to new evidence.

When cases are sent up the hospital chain for hospital quality program review, it often takes weeks to months for the case to return. The hospital may require that records documenting hospital committee output be kept in a separate place and may be difficult to access. The program needs to negotiate with the hospital and method by which the reviewers can see the output of the hospital PI process. Otherwise, it will appear that the case was sent to the hospital and then disappeared into a black hole. Since cases that are referred to the hospital often are serious, it would look quite bad for all if the final analysis of serious opportunities for improvement are in an area where they cannot be accessed.

Your PI plan as well as your PI manual (if one exists) as well as your PI program policies and procedures should also be available for the reviewers.

Open Loops

Not every opportunity improvement gets loop closure. In fact, some problems cannot be fixed. Reviewers will be concerned when they see that very few opportunities undergo loop closure but experienced trauma directors understand that some loop closure is extremely difficult if not impossible. As an example, let us say adverse events arise from the fact that your emergency department is five floors away and 500 yards away from the operating requiring long transport times for emergent patients where complications occur. It is highly unlikely that your hospital will move either its emergency department or its operating rooms in response to a PI concern. You merely need to document that you discuss this and that you try to formulate corrective actions that could ameliorate the problem knowing that permanently fixing the problem is impossible unless the hospital is rebuilt.

For open loops, it is important that the program documents the effort that was put into closing the loop, and if obstructions were with specific people, documentation of these discussions can be helpful. Very few hospitals are subservient to the trauma program, so there will be instances in every hospital with the trauma program that cannot get its way. You merely need to have documentation that you expended reasonable effort to overcome resistance. A reviewer should not expect that every problem can be solved but can expect that you do not just throw your hands up in the air after expending minimal effort to correct a serious issue.

I am often asked how long corrective action plans need to be audited. There is no really good answer to this question. We are well aware that having continued auditing for long periods of time of multiple corrective action plans would consume all the time of the program. For certain corrective action plans where simple data abstraction can demonstrate compliance, this should be done until the process is stable. A measurement period of three to six months is the norm. If a corrective action plan requires extensive chart review to determine compliance, the program can simply say that they will assume that the plan is in place unless another event occurs. While this is not perfect and cannot be used for everything, reviewers will understand that auditing is not possible in all cases. However, the reviewers will be concerned when they see the problem keeps cropping up over and over even though a beautiful corrective action plan was created. Remember the loop is not closed merely by the creation of the corrective action plan. You must demonstrate in some way that the corrective action plan was implemented and that it addressed the problem. I realize this is a somewhat unclear explanation of what is needed in auditing these plans, and reasonable effort will go a long way toward demonstrating that you did your best.

Reference

1. Young JS. Trauma Centers: a quick guide: Springer Nature; 2020.

Chapter 14
Performance Improvement Case Studies

Documents and Slides

Below are examples of the agenda for an MDPI meeting, and many of the documents we us in our PI program.

MDPI Agenda
- Open forum
- Attendance roll call
- Equipment on helipad(s)
- Blood supply/FAST/MTP (Fig. 14.1). Demonstration of new MTP cooler

Fig. 14.1 New MTP cooler

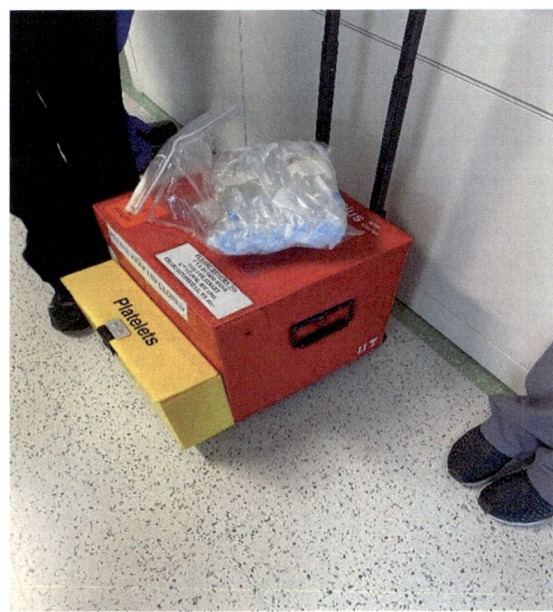

- ED/trauma graphs
- Trauma continuum of care during COVID crisis
- COVID screenings/testing
- Imaging guidelines
- Transfer changes
- Liaison reports

These are the blank forms that we currently use for PI activities:

The Trauma Alert EMS follow-up form (Fig. 14.2) is sent back to the transporting EMS agencies as soon as possible after admission.

Figure 14.3 is our mortality review template. This template is used to organize the mortality review process and provides a framework for review of the case.

Figure 14.4 is a template of the feedback letter we send to treating clinicians, or department heads to communicate our findings from our PI meetings. This is included in the formal PI record for review by site visitors. It is important to ensure these letters are received and read by the addressee. This is usually done with an affirmative response from that person that is also included in the PI record.

Figure 14.5 is a blank template of our MDPI minutes to demonstrate the necessary elements.

The following are examples of slides from MDPI where corrective action plans and audits are presented. Figure 14.6 demonstrates the loop closure for our continued effort to revise our massive transfusion system. This pathway is the product of several years of PI activity.

EMS - Trauma Alert Feedback

Privileged & Confidential Quality Assurance Document under Virginia Code Section 8.01 - 581.17.

Incident Information						
Incident Date:			Incident #:			
EMS Agency:			Method of Transport:			
Patient Information						
Patient Age:			Patient Gender:			
Mechanism of Injury:						
EMS Report						
Time on Scene:		Transport Time:		Notification to Medcom:	(Goal <15 mins)	
Type of Spinal Motion Restriction:	☐ C-Collar ☐ Long Board		☐ None, Reason:			
IV/IO Placed Prior to Arrival (if indicated):	☐ Yes ☐ No		Pain Management Utilized:			
Assessment Notes						
Hospital Course and Findings						
Trauma Alert Level: ☐ Alpha ☐ Beta ☐ Gamma						
Reason for Trauma Alert:						
BP:	HR:	RR:	SPO2:	ETCO2:	GCS:	Temp:
Injuries:						
Hospital Course:						
Performance Improvement Follow Up:						

Please contact me if you have any further questions on this patient.

Fig. 14.2 Trauma Alert EMS follow-up form

Figure 14.7 demonstrates our ongoing audit of emergency department dwell times. This is a permanent audit filter for our program and allows us to identify changes in throughput that may not be evident without measurement.

Figure 14.8 demonstrates our ongoing efforts to ensure that the temperature of new trauma patients is measured during their resuscitation. This was the result of adverse events related to hypothermia.

Cases

Below are a series of fabricated PI cases based on the hundreds I have analyzed as a site reviewer. I have split the cases into three sections: case narrative, description of PI process, and a critique. My comments center on the quality and

Name/MRN: Death Date:

Patient Information			
Name:	MRN:	Age:	Gender:

Case Information				
Date of Service:	Date of Death:		Site of Death:	
Prehospital:			Transfer Hospital:	
Alert Status:	Alert Notice:		ED Attending:	
Trauma MD:	Admin Attending:		Admin Service:	
Initial Vitals:				
Comorbidities:				
MOI:				
Injuries:				
Complications:				
Summary:				
LOS:	ICU Days:	ISS:	POS:	RTS:

Initial Assessment of Preventability – MD Review	
Reviewer Name: Choose an item.	Date of Review: Date

☐ Mortality without opportunity for improvement
☐ Anticipated mortality (or preventability of death difficult to discern) with opportunity for improvement
☐ Unanticipated mortality with opportunity for improvement

Initial Assessment of Opportunity for Improvement

Who do you want further input from (i.e. Ortho, ED...)? Please specify question needed addressed

Fig. 14.3 Mortality review template

Name/MRN: Death Date:

PI Coordinator Investigation Notes	
PI Coordinator Name: Valerie Quick, MSN, RN	**Date of Review:** Date
Prehospital Summary: Click here to enter text.	
ED Summary	
Hospital Summary	
Timeline	
Complication Review	
Co-Morbid Review	
Pertinent Labs	
Recommended Preventability and Opportunities for Improvement	

Issue	Description	Primary Classification (Impact, Type, Domain, Cause)	Action

Fig. 14.3 (continued)

Name/MRN: Death Date:

Action Items			
Topic	Sent to	Date Requested	Response

Autopsy Information

Was an autopsy offered? ☐Yes ☐No   *Was an autopsy granted?* ☐Yes ☐No   *ME Case:* ☐Yes ☐No

Autopsy Findings

UBL Meeting Discussions

Date : Date

Discussion Notes

Be Safe Review

Date : Date

Notes

Trauma Meeting Discussions

Friday Trauma Service Conference	*Date :* Date
Discussion Notes	
Surgery M&M	*Date :* Date

Fig. 14.3 (continued)

Name/MRN: Death Date:

Discussion Notes	
Tuesday Trauma Divisional Meetings	*Date(s) :* Date
Discussion Notes	
Corrective Actions	
Ready for MDPI: ☐Yes ☐No	*Date :* Date

MDPI
Date : Date
Discussion Notes
MDPI Preventability Assessment
☐ Mortality without opportunity for improvement ☐ Anticipated mortality (or preventability of death difficult to discern) with opportunity for improvement ☐ Unanticipated mortality with opportunity for improvement
Determination
☐ System Related   ☐ Missed injury ☐ Disease Related   ☐ Technique Issue ☐ Provider Related   ☐ Communication ☐ Protocol Related   ☐ Other
Opportunities for Improvement
Corrective Actions
☐ Not necessary   ☐ PIPS Team Project ☐ Trend/track similar occurrences   ☐ Hospital System PI ☐ Education   ☐ Develop/Revise Guideline ☐ Counseling   ☐ Other
Further Details

Fig. 14.3 (continued)

Name/MRN: Death Date:

Final Determination
Final Preventability Assignment
☐ Mortality without opportunity for improvement ☐ Anticipated mortality (or preventability of death difficult to discern) with opportunity for improvement ☐ Unanticipated mortality with opportunity for improvement
Opportunities for Improvement
Corrective Actions
Loop Closure
Date Closed : Click here to enter a date.

Trauma Registry Information

Fig. 14.3 (continued)

Date

Re: Click here to enter text.

Dear Click here to enter text.,

At the date meeting of the Trauma program MDPI the committee reviewed the death of
name (MRN: MRN). The death was determined to be *Choose an item.*. We write to
provide feedback on what was discussed at the meeting and have attached
the information presented with any recommended actions or comments.

On behalf of our entire trauma team, please allow me to thank you for your ongoing
engagement and thoughtful care of our mutual patients. I would also like to offer you
the opportunity to contact me if there is any part of this encounter or message you
would like to discuss.

Fig. 14.4 MDPI feedback letter

Patient Information

Case Information

Opportunities for Improvement: *Last Name (MRN)*

Issue	Description	Primary Classification (Impact, Type, Domain, Cause)

Recommended Action:	

Anonymous Survey Comments:

- Click here to enter text.

Preventability Question	Respondents
Anticipated Mortality without OFI	
Anticipated Mortality with OFI	
Unanticipated Mortality with OFI	

Final Determination: Choose an item.

Fig. 14.4 (continued)

TRAUMA MULTI-DISCIPLINARY PERFORMANCE IMPROVEMENT (MDPI)
Date:

Agenda Item	Discussion	Action	Responsible Party
Open Forum			
Attendance			
Mortality with no OFI			
Mortality with OFIs – Case Discussions			
Adjournment			

Attached Documents:

- Qualtrics Questionnaire
- MDPI Slides

Fig. 14.5 MDPI minutes template

ORDERING BLOOD PRODUCTS
3 PATHWAYS
University of Virginia Health System Effective March 24, 2020

PATHWAY TURNAROUND TIME	ORDER	CLINICAL GUIDELINES	PRODUCTS	DELIVERY SYSTEM
ROUTINE < 30 minutes if antibodies	**EPIC**	✓ HEMODYNAMICALLY STABLE PATIENT	**AS ORDERED**	**TUBE SYSTEM**
FASTBLOOD 3 + 3 < 15 minutes	CALL 4-2012 TO *ACTIVATE* FastBlood 3+3 NOT RECURRENT "ONE AND DONE"	✓ URGENT NEED ✓ ESTIMATED/PREDICTED ACUTE BLOOD LOSS > 750 mL ✓ HEART RATE > 100 bpm ✓ SYSTOLIC BP < 100 mm Hg ✓ ABC TRAUMA SCORE 0 OR 1	3 PLASMA 3 RBC	**ALL PRODUCTS IN ONE *IGLOO* COOLER** Delivered by Transportation
MTP **MASSIVE TRANSFUSION PROTOCOL** < 15 minutes to first cooler 5 + 5 + 1	CALL 4-2012 TO *ACTIVATE* MTP **RECURRING** CLINICAL TEAM DECISION; CHECK THE BOX ON THE ACTIVATION FORM WITH EACH COOLER DELIVERY ✓ CONTINUE every 15 minutes ✓ HOLD – clinical team calls the blood bank when ready for more blood ✓ DEACTIVATE - stops the cooler delivery Blood bank will auto-deactivate after 2 hours of inactivity	✓ EMERGENT NEED ✓ ESTIMATED/ PREDICTED ACUTE BLOOD LOSS> 1500 mL ✓ HEART RATE > 120 bpm ✓ SYSTOLIC BP < 90 mm Hg ✓ ABC TRAUMA SCORE 2 OR GREATER	5 PLASMA 5 RBC 1 PLATELET 1 CRYO BLOOD BANK CALLS TO DETERMINE NEED FOR CRYO WITH 2ⁿᵈ COOLER CRYO CONTINUES WITH EVERY OTHER COOLER	**ALL PRODUCTS IN ONE *MAXPLUS* COOLER** Delivered by Transportation

CALL 4-2012 TO ACTIVATE Fast Blood or MTP – Initiates the Fast Blood or MTP
Blood Bank will begin to process blood products and prepare for delivery via transportation
CALL 4-2012 TO DEACTIVATE MTP – Stops the MTP Process
Blood Bank stops processing products for MTP
CALL 4-2012 WHEN PATIENT CHANGES LOCATION
Alerts transportation of location change for expedient cooler delivery

Give the Call Center the following information
✓ Patient Name or Trauma Name
✓ Patient Age (under or over 12 years)
✓ Medical Record Number (MRN)
✓ Ordering Doctor and PIC #
✓ Location of Patient

Fig. 14.6 Blood ordering pathway

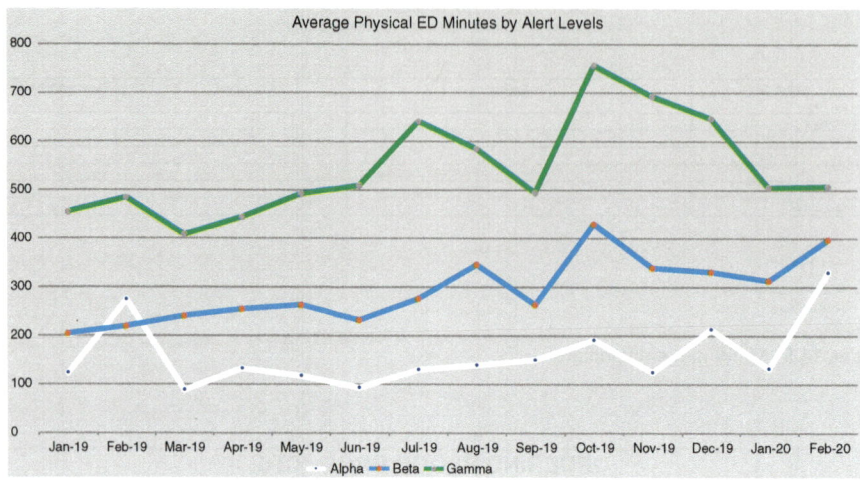

Fig. 14.7 ED dwell time graphs

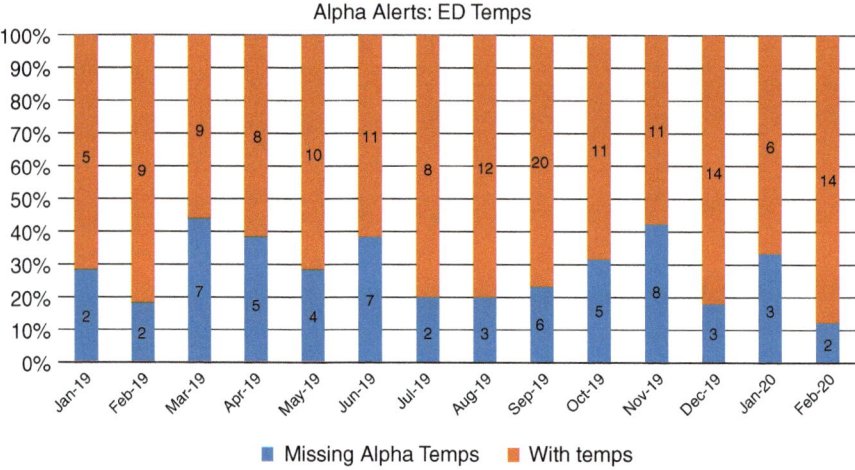

Fig. 14.8 ED temperature record

appropriateness of the PI review and actions. These case descriptions do not in any way represent the gold standard of how to address these issues, but these cases represent a cross section of PI problems and how they were addressed. This section also demonstrates the way that reviewers break down and assess cases.

Note: *ACS site reviewers will always check if the prehospital patient record is available, and they will audit every emergency department flow sheet to review documentation and note the trauma surgeon arrival time (especially in highest-level activations). This is noted in some of the cases so that the reader is reminded that these documents must be available.*

Missed Injuries

Case Narrative: This is a 60-year-old female pedestrian struck isolated to leg injury. The patient was a consult in the ED and was admitted to the trauma service. Orthopedics was the primary consulting service and they evaluated the patient rapidly. The patient was taken to the operating room the following day for external fixation of a tib/fib open fracture.

Postoperatively, the patient had intermittent agitation that was attributed to a long history of ethanol abuse. On postoperative day 2, the patient was given a diet. The following day, the patient's urine output dropped and respiratory function declined. The trauma team evaluated the patient and diagnosed abdominal compartment syndrome and the patient taken to the OR. The patient was found to have a large necrotic colon and underwent a subtotal colectomy. The patient declined postoperatively. The family refused dialysis and the patient was made comfort care.

Description of PI Process: The case underwent initial and secondary review and went to surgical M&M and the trauma program PI conference. On review and discussion with radiology, the PI process concluded that on re-review of the patient's initial studies by independent radiologists, no injury to the colon could be identified. The largest opportunity for improvement was variability in the ETOH withdrawal process. A guideline for adult alcohol withdrawal was reviewed and re-educated.

Critique:
Dealing with missed injuries can be a true test of a program's self-reflection. No surgeon likes to admit mistakes and that goes for every other specialty (especially radiology), though the independent review of the films without providing information about the outcomes was excellent. However, there was at least 24 hours where the patient was acting "squirrely" and the presumption was that the patient was withdrawing from alcohol, when they were actually becoming septic. The program did not identify this until multiple organ failure began. This is definitely an OFI and should have been investigated. Though they did adequate follow-up and loop closure on alcohol withdrawal education, that was a contributing factor but not the root cause of the patient's demise. The PI program should have delved into the exact data from the time the patient became agitated, to the point where it was determined that the patient needed to go to the operating room. In a university setting, the root cause of these types of errors of omission are usually an inexperienced nurse and physician who both make incorrect assumptions and allowed too much time to elapse before escalating the issue.

There are many potential corrective actions for that issue including the charge nurse rounds on every shift to insure that subtle clues are not being missed, or setting guidelines such that new onset of agitation always triggers a more involved examination since it can mask a wide variety of serious problems.

If this type of problem was found in multiple PI charts, then the reviewer would likely feel that the program does superficial analysis and would likely award a weakness or possibly a deficiency if the pattern was consistent.

Failure to Rescue and Escalation

Case Narrative: This is a 67-year-old female who fell down a flight of stairs. The patient was a direct admit and did not pass through the emergency department but was admitted directly to the SICU. The principal diagnosis was central cord syndrome identified on MRI. The patient's initial vital signs were stable. Neurosurgery was consulted and the patient was taken to the operating room for a laminectomy and cervical fusion.

Postoperatively: Two days later, the patient developed hypoxia and required intubation. MRI revealed a spinal cord infarct and neck hematoma. The patient continued to do poorly neurologically and a trach and PEG were performed. The patient progressed to renal failure. Care was withdrawn.

Description of PI Process: The opportunity for improvement revolved around the unplanned return to OR and neurosurgery complications. The patient did not have a pulmonary embolism. An opportunity for improvement that was identified was that the patient's change in neurosurgery exam was not rapidly communicated to the neurosurgery team; thus, the bleed may have been intervened upon earlier. In discussion and documentation, it was unclear whether there was a delay because the patient initially presented with respiratory decompensation and not with new neurologic deficits.

Critique: Postoperatively, the bleed was deemed non-preventable. There was a discussion of the delay in notification which was proper, but due to the respiratory crash, neurosurgery was called as soon as the patient was awake enough after intubation to obtain a neurologic exam. The possibility that the intubation itself may have led to the complication was not discussed, but the patient required intubation so it is unclear that could have been prevented. Overall this is an acceptable PI process as long as documentation was adequate.

The Impact of Learners on Outcomes, Airway Management

Case Narrative: This is a 53-year-old male s/p propane tank explosion. The trauma flow sheet was reviewed and the trauma surgeon was present on arrival. Patient arrived with 20–25% TBSA burn with copious secretions. The surgery chief resident attempted intubation and was unsuccessful. Then multiple attempts were made with significant drops in saturations. A surgical airway was performed, but the patient had an asystolic arrest coincident with securing the airway. The patient underwent a vigorous resuscitation and was stabilized after ~40 minutes. The patient then underwent a trauma workup, and various non-life-threatening injuries were identified. The patient did not regain any mental status, and the family withdrew care after a long hospital course.

Description of PI Process: The case was presented at trauma QA committee. A primary issue was that the surgical airway equipment could not be produced in the middle of the situation. This case led to a complete reorganization of the equipment and supplies in both trauma bays. Other airway adjuncts were also thoroughly discussed. The case was also discussed in the main hospital clinical quality management committee. The corrective actions were the equipment reorganization and an EM faculty educated the EM and surgery residents/attendings on emergency airway algorithms. Auditing of equipment and supplies are done on a regular basis.

Comment: They reacted to this case rapidly, and instituted both organizational and educational corrective actions rapidly: good PI response to an unfortunate case. However this case raises an interesting point, should the surgical resident have been responsible for the airway? The vast majority of hospitals let EM or anesthesia control the airway, especially in high-risk situations. The root cause of the outcome was not necessarily the lack of equipment but a lack of expertise on the part of the person performing the procedure. Should a surgery resident have been responsible for airway management and a case that was clearly high-risk? There was no evidence that this was discussed. There are certainly no criteria in the document that are used for site visits that prohibit the surgical resident from controlling the airway; many reviewers would not think this is in the best interest of the patient. But surgeons who do feel that airway management should be part of their skills, usually feel very strongly about this (because they would likely face a great deal of resistance in their organization) and likely would not respond well to the reviewer objecting to this. An experienced reviewer would treat this like any other airway misadventure. Is it common for the person tasked with placing the airway to be unsuccessful? They could feel that the program was not diligent if they did not at least ask the question as to whether the success rate of surgery residents and airway management was audited.

They can get this question from several angles. They can ask the program to show them how many surgical airways were placed in the emergency department since this should be part of their registry. From that information they could ask that audits be performed to see who was most commonly performing airway management in those cases where surgical airway was needed. It would not be appropriate for the reviewer to simply say that surgery residents should not be managing the airway in trauma patients since this is not part of our criteria. However, it is not unreasonable for them to say that any missed airway in the emergency department should initiate a thorough review of intubations success rates and action if the rates were found to be low.

Unstable Patients at Referring Hospitals

Case Narrative: This is a 45-year-old female with a self-inflicted GSW to the abdomen. She was taken to a referring facility and then transferred. This was a trauma alpha activation, and the attending was present prior to arrival. The patient was taken to the OR within 30 minutes of arrival. The patient underwent a colon resection, nephrectomy, and colectomy and was returned to the OR 5 days later for a second look and no obvious issue was identified. She progressively developed respiratory failure and underwent tracheostomy. An intra-abdominal abscess was drained percutaneously on hospital day 15. She also had further septic complications and eventually succumbed.

Description of PI Process: Multiple PI filters were triggered and investigated with excellent documentation. The case was discussed in their PI conference and it was felt that the patient's renal failure was not expected, and the development of the abscess was indirect evidence of operative issues. The counseling was done among the attending involved at the meeting. All of this is well documented.

Critique: Excellent performance improvement was performed in this case, and there was excellent documentation. One possible avenue up for investigation would be to ensure that the actions at the referring hospital were appropriate. This is another very delicate area for trauma programs. As regionalization of trauma care has improved the ability of nondesignated trauma, centers to perform any interventional trauma care has decreased. An important question that could arise would be if this patient had a systolic blood pressure of 60 mmHg prior to transfer, and the transport time was 60 minutes, with the patient have survived to reach the trauma center? In those cases what would the referring hospital do? It would be attracted to say that they should take the patient to the operating room, control obvious pleading, and packed the abdomen prior to transfer. However in reality, many of these hospitals do not have the capability to take the patient from the emergency department to the operating room within 60 minutes, and are not required to. By telling the referring hospital that they must do this, the trauma center may actually be delaying the care of the patient. Therefore, it is important for trauma directors to have situational awareness of the capabilities of their most frequent referring hospitals. If the hospital did have sufficient capability to take the patient to the operating room rapidly, there should be discussion with the surgical leadership of that hospital as to what could be done in certain unstable cases.

New Technologies

This is an 25-year-old male involved in an all-terrain vehicle crash. This was a highest-level activation and the trauma surgeon was present prior to arrival. The EMS run sheet was available for review. The patient had a patent airway on arrival and GCS of 4. The patient was grossly unstable hemodynamically on arrival. The patient was intubated. Ultrasound of the abdomen (FAST) was negative, and an aortic occlusion catheter (REBOA) was placed but the balloon was not inflated. The patient was found to have a liver laceration with active extravasation. Pulses were lost in the operating room and CPR was begun, along with massive transfusions. The patient recovered vital signs. The patient's abdomen was packed and the patient prepared for angiography when the patient coded again and could not be resuscitated.

Description of PI Process: Issues focused on whether the patient should have had a thoracotomy on arrest, why REBOA was not inflated until after arrest, and that the FAST was false negative with the large hemoperitoneum found in OR. There was loop closure with education in the placement of REBOA.

Critique: The use of new technology and techniques including REBOA can be an area of discussion in a site review. This applies to other technologies and techniques such as elastography (ROTEM) and operative pelvic packing. Since most new technologies and techniques are not universally accepted, it is quite possible your site reviewer will not be a fan. An appropriate site reviewer should not tell the program that the use of a certain technology or technique is wrong. They should always be looking at this from a PI perspective. The proper question would be how often is the technology being used? How did the outcomes of patients who receive this technology compare to similar patients before it was implemented? For a technique such as REBOA, what are the success rates in placement? How often has it been used? What is the required training? Are there any delays created by the use of the technique? These are the types of questions that a mature PI program would be asking itself before accepting any new technique or technology. Naturally trauma care must improve as we gain more knowledge, but the PI program should make certain that the introduction of something new does not worsen outcomes.

Airway Management

Case Narrative: This is a 78-year-old male who sustained a GSW to the face. The EMS run sheet was available for review. This was a highest-level activation and the trauma surgeon was present prior to arrival. A rapid sequence intubation was attempted and was unsuccessful. Anesthesia indicated that they were able to move air, but the patient desaturated and became bradycardic. A cricothyroidotomy was performed, but the patient went into cardiac arrest and could not be resuscitated.

Description of PI Process: It was felt there was adequate IV access and that the surgical airway was performed correctly by the attendings. There were questions raised as to whether sedation should have been given with tenuous airway, and whether awake fiberoptic intubation should have been done. There is documentation from the chief of anesthesia on these points, and it was felt fiberoptic was not possible due to bleeding. The patient underwent induction and received no sedation. The autopsy was reviewed and it demonstrated an extremely distorted airway.

Critique: Sometimes bad outcomes are unavoidable even in the best trauma centers. Any time a patient dies from airway management the program must be very critical of itself. A red flag to reviewers is a cursory examination of the case where an airway disaster occurs. This is the reason why I will often review death charts from the anticipated mortality without OFI group. Many week trauma centers will place cases in this category that would be salvageable in other hospitals. For instance, a case where a patient has a gunshot wound to the brain with brain matter evident would certainly be expected to be an anticipated death, but what if an airway cannot be obtained, IV access cannot be obtained, or a CT scanner was not available? It is important that even in cases where the outcome is certain, the PI program should do a thorough review and should engage when they find areas in the patient's treatment there were suboptimal. For instance, in this case, I do have concerns as to whether a supraglottic airway could have been used. Many site reviewers have personal experiences that differentiate them from other reviewers. For instance, in my case, I have extensive experience with EMS and supraglottic airways are commonly used in the prehospital setting enters rarely used in the hospital setting. In a review of the case within airway management problem, the PI program should look at the case from the perspective of the patient. Would a patient rather have a less optimal airway in place and been ventilated, or have no airway established using traditional tools. This sort of criticism would certainly not rise to the level of a weakness or deficiency, but consistent evidence that the PI program is not doing thorough reviews in cases where mortality was almost certain can indicate an inadequate PI program.

Patients with Life-Threatening Injuries Who Die in the Operating Room

This is a 39-year-old female with a GSW to the chest and abdomen. The trauma attending was present, and the patient was taken directly to the OR. The patient underwent thoracotomy, laparotomy, cardiac injury repair, repair of the stomach, splenectomy, wedge resection of right lung, hepatic resection, and cardiac massage. The patient succumbed in the OR.

Description of PI Process: Case was discussed and no OFIs were identified.

Critique: This certainly seems like appropriate care for this patient. It is highly unlikely that a significant opportunity for improvement would be identified. But in cases where the patient dies of hemorrhage, a thorough review is needed. Stopping hemorrhage is the sine qua non of trauma centers. To fail in this primary mission should warrant introspection. In these types of cases, a few areas of investigation are indicated. Was prehospital care optimal? (Was time at the scene too long?) Was blood available in the emergency department on arrival? Was the operating room ready when the patient arrived? Did the surgeon and the anesthesiologist have adequate assistance during the procedure? Was the massive transfusion protocol followed? The PI program must look at every case is an opportunity to improve, even if it felt the actions of the team were heroic. A thorough investigation of the individual processes in patient care can reveal ways to improve the system for the next patient.

Here is a similar case with the different PI review:

Case Narrative: A 41-year-old female presents after a motorcycle crash. On arrival of EMS, the patient is talking, spitting up blood, and complaining of dyspnea. The patient was orotracheally intubated prehospital for airway protection. In the emergency department, the FAST was positive and the patient remained hypotensive despite two units of blood. A CXR was performed and patient was taken to the OR. The patient lost her pulse in the OR, and a thoracotomy was performed and the aorta was cross clamped. The patient was found to have a Grade V liver injury and a large retroperitoneal hematoma. On exploration, an IVC hole was found. The patient succumbed in the OR.

PI: This case was reviewed in the weekly meeting. The PI program reviewed several processes of care. The EMS crew spent 40 minutes at the scene prior to transport, and this was felt to be excessive. From review of the record and discussion with the agency, the delay in transport was attributed to the time taken to place IVs and obtaining airway. Feedback was provided to the EMS agency that in patients with this level of instability, all procedures should be performed en route to the hospital. The patient is bleeding to death and every minute is precious. There was a close loop with EMS agency in the form of an educational presentation that was given as an in-service on unstable trauma patients. The time in the ED before transfer was ~25 minutes, and this was felt to be acceptable. The massive transfusion protocol (MTP) was activated prior to arrival, and several coolers of blood were in the ED on arrival. The operative record was reviewed with the anesthesia liaison, and it was felt that due to the time of day (4 AM) there were not sufficient anesthesia personnel available. A process was instituted where if information is obtained indicating a patient is unstable and will very likely go to the operating room, the backup anesthesiologist is automatically notified and is expected to drive to the hospital. This loop was closed. Overall, the case was classified as possibly preventable due to exsanguination.

Critique: There are many parts of this PI process that indicate a very mature trauma center. The review was thorough and dealt with all critical areas. There was loop closure and every opportunity that was identified, and finally because the patient examining the case is classified as possibly preventable. This program feels that any patient who arrives at their center alive who dies of bleeding is a potentially preventable death. This indicates a program is extremely critical of its own care and is providing the best care possible.

Life-Threatening Thoracic Trauma

Case Narrative: This is a 45-year-old male patient found unresponsive and was found with a GSW to the chest. The patient began to awaken en route. The EMS run sheet was available. This was a highest-level activation, and the trauma surgeon was present prior to arrival. The patient was initially hypotensive and FAST was negative. CXR showed a hemothorax on the left with a shift of the mediastinum. A chest tube was inserted and 1100 cc returned. The patient remained hypotensive and follow-up chest film did not show resolution of hemothorax. The patient was taken to OR within 40 minutes of arrival and was in extremis at that point. Thoracotomy was performed. There was a hilar injury identified and a large injury to the right ventricle. The patient could not be resuscitated.

Description of PI Process: The time to OR of 35 minutes was identified as an opportunity for improvement. The case was discussed at M&M, and peer review and education were performed with the trauma attending. The presentation at M&M, and the education that was given on penetrating cardiac and thoracic trauma, was included with the chart.

Critique: In trauma centers without a great deal of penetrating trauma to the chest, an operative chest case is uncommon. The vast majority of thoracic injuries are disposed of with a chest tube and pain control. However, the center must be ready to perform life-saving thoracic surgery any time of the day or night. But in most centers, there is not a thoracic surgeon available immediately, especially in the night and evening hours. A good question to ask the team is what would occur if the patient needed immediate thoracic surgery and no thoracic surgeon was immediately available. Were the trauma surgeons comfortable with performing a thoracotomy or sternotomy? After performing a sternotomy, what would they do next? Would they open the pericardium, and place sutures in the heart laceration? These are not questions that would lead to a weakness or deficiency, but it does give the reviewer insight into how that trauma center functions with less common injuries.

Another disturbing problem I have seen in a variety of community hospitals is an unwillingness for thoracic surgery to give up any of their practice. I have seen centers where trauma medical directors had to go through months of arguments in order for their trauma fellowship-trained general surgeons to place chest tubes. While the American College of Surgeons does not mandate the trauma surgeons must place chest tubes, they do mandate that life-saving treatment needs to be immediately available and if chest tubes are common enough that the thoracic surgeon needs to be in house, I can bet that they will no longer demand putting chest tubes. In centers such as this the reviewers will often ask for charts where chest tubes were placed in order to evaluate for delays and complications.

An insight into the quality of the trauma center can be gained from a case like this. I have seen centers where any central thoracic injury initiates a call to the cardiothoracic surgeon on call and the perfusionist. I have also seen systems where a fully equipped thoracic trauma case card is always available in the operating room with all the necessary equipment to perform any operation in the chest. These are the sorts of things that would lead the team to award strengths during their visit, and a large number of strengths can offset some low-intensity weaknesses.

Getting back to this case, it would be interesting to read the center's PI analysis of the 35 minutes that were spent in the emergency department before taking the patient to the operating room. Actually 35 minutes is pretty good with respect to getting a patient in the operating room from patient arrival in the emergency department. For a program to feel that a 35 minute time between arrival in the ED and arrival in the operating room was excessive would indicate a program that it takes a long hard look at all the care providers and is very self-critical, which is a positive.

Adverse Events

Case Narrative: This is an 88-year-old male in a rollover MVC with paraplegia at scene. This was a highest-level activation, but there is missing documentation of the presence of the attending surgeon. But there is a contemporaneous note from the trauma fellow. The patient was hemodynamically unstable in the ED and was emergently intubated. The patient was found to have a C3 fracture, pulmonary injury, and

L3 fracture. The patient had delayed fixation due to severe respiratory failure. The fixation was eventually done; the patient received a tracheostomy and feeding access. During turning in CT scan, the tracheostomy was dislodged and there was difficulty re-establishing the airway. The patient coded and could not be resuscitated.

Description of PI Process: The case was reviewed. It was felt that a longer trache tube should have been used, but there was disagreement with that conclusion among the attendings. The patient could not be intubated from above. Nursing issues were also addressed. Education and discussion were the methods of loop closure.

Critique: There are many issues in this case. Starting from the beginning, trauma program should examine the case closely when the patient requires intubation immediately on arrival in the trauma bay. The question that comes to mind is, why was not the patient's airway control in the prehospital setting? This is an important question in that some patients can suffer severe deterioration in a short period of time if they require airway control and it is not provided. This is the type of case where a discussion with the EMS liaison can be valuable. This is also an issue where the trauma center can provide education and training.

Second, there was no documentation of the presence of the attending trauma surgeon, but the reviewer took the extra time to read additional notes and found that the appropriate personnel were present upon the arrival of the patient. This does demonstrate how important it is for the trauma program to go through all the charts that they are in the present to find problems and be ready with answers.

But the most important part of this case is the dislodgement of the tracheostomy and the patient's subsequent death. This is the most serious adverse event that any program can encounter. It represents a salvageable patient who is recovering who then dies from a preventable complication. The actions in the CT scanner should be reviewed carefully, and the PI personnel should conduct personal interviews with the clinicians who were present. As we all know, these types of situations are frantic, and a good outcome requires strong leadership, the availability of appropriate personnel, and cool heads. The program should go minute by minute through the care provided from leaving the clinical care unit until the patient's death. What personnel were with the patient? What equipment was available? Were there any problems with the tracheostomy before the patient left the ICU? Was the CT scan even indicated? How was the tracheostomy secured? What were the steps taken once it was realized that the patient lost their airway?

The reason for this seemingly paranoid analysis is that airway misadventures are tragic. They often lead to either the patient's death or serious neurological devastation. They also commonly occur in patients on their way to recovery. Thus, the program should show great enthusiasm after one of these events to ensure that the same event does not occur again. To do this may include placing equipment in radiology for airway management, working with the hospital to provide surgical airway kits in various locations, training and education by all care providers and what to do when a patient loses their airway, and review of the steps that should be taken immediately whenever an airway is lost. Often in these cases, trying to achieve a perfect solution obviates a good solution. What you need in these situations is merely to maintain oxygenation and ventilation. If you can do that you can calm down and wait until you gather the right personnel in the right equipment to obtain a more definitive solution. I also realize that some of these cases are unsalvageable, but that does not relieve the program of the responsibility to take an extremely close look at these types of cases.

Dislodged Gastrostomy Tubes

Case Narrative: A 22-year-old female found unresponsive with a washing machine on top of her. The EMS run sheet is on the chart. This was a highest-level activation, and the trauma surgeon was present 11 minutes after arrival. She was intubated at a referring hospital, and her GCS was 8 T on arrival. CT of the head revealed a large right-sided EDH, and she was taken to the OR for craniotomy within 27 minutes of arrival. She underwent a craniotomy and evacuation. Her postoperative course was complicated by seizures and she was transferred to the primary supervision of the neurosurgeons. On hospital day 21, she became difficult to ventilate and suffered a cardiac arrest. She was found to have a firm abdomen and intra-abdominal pressures of 36. A bedside laparotomy was performed and a displaced gastrostomy tube was found. The patient dies the following day.

Description of PI Process: The case was extensively reviewed. It was concluded there was a delay in identification of the dislodged PEG, that the laparotomy should have been performed in the OR, and that the securing of the PEG may have been too tight leading to the dislodgement. Corrective actions included presentation at both resident conferences and critical care conferences with specific education regarding signs of PEG displacement and securing of PEG at proper this was a highest-level activation (>3 cm).

Critique: This is an example of a case with excellent discussion and investigation. The reader may not understand why I create a separate case for dislodged gastrostomy tubes. However any trauma surgeon knows that this complication is not rare, unfortunately, and can have a devastating effect. Most trauma patients in the intensive care unit have firm abdomens, and it can be very difficult to detect subtle changes over the course of 12-hour shifts. Invariably dislodged gastrostomy tubes are not identified until the patient become septic. Once that occurs the chance of a good outcome drops significantly.

This program did an excellent job of creating an overall protocol for workup of fever and SIRS in the patient with a recent PEG and specifications for securing PEG could have been added. The only thing missing could be an ongoing audit of whether PEG tubes are being secured as specified, but that is not critical.

Optimal Case

This is a 52-year-old male who presented with multiple GSW to arms and center of back. Per EMS, the patient was found in arrest and had return of circulation by the time he arrived at the trauma center. This was a highest-level activation, and the trauma surgeon was present prior to arrival. The patient arrived and was lethargic and was immediately intubated. Two chest tubes were placed and there was massive blood return from the left tube. The patient lost pulses and CPR was begun. A thoracotomy was performed; there was a massive left hemothorax and no tamponade. FAST was positive and patient taken to OR. In the OR, a laparotomy, sternotomy, lung resection, and cholecystectomy were performed and an atriocaval shunt was placed, but the patient succumbed.

Description of PI Process: Case review concluded that the time required for intubation was extremely long, and there was a similar delay in provision of blood products. The provider was counseled and the case was presented at their video review conference.

Critique: I present this case as an example of optimal care and PI. On initial review, the care here was excellent and the patient was unsalvageable. Many programs will look at a case like this in relegated to their bin of anticipated mortalities without opportunity for improvement. This program did not do that. They delved deeply into the case and were able to perform video review of the resuscitation. During the review of the resuscitation, they were disappointed by the amount of time it took to ready the patient for intubation, thus delaying the patient's transport to the operating room. Though it is certain this made absolutely no difference in the patient's outcome, it is a potential area for improvement that may save a patient in the future. The ability to do video review is an incredibly powerful PI tool. It is unfortunate that due to legal issues and HIPAA concerns, most trauma centers have given up on doing video recording of resuscitations. It is likely that video review at this center serves to consistently improve the conduct of their resuscitations and is a powerful educational tool. Since video review is not available at most trauma centers, the only substitute is a contemporaneous debriefing of the resuscitation team once the patient has been brought to a stable area. This will preserve fragile information and allow people to discuss the problems they faced and come up with solutions.

Pediatric

This is a 7-year-old male brought in by EMS after being struck while riding a bike without a helmet. EMS documented fixed and dilated pupils on arrival and agonal breathing. The patient was intubated at the scene. The patient was initially a second-level activation, but was upgraded to a highest level on arrival. An intraosseous catheter was placed in the field. On arrival due to low saturations, the patient was re-intubated by anesthesia. A cervical collar was not in place and was placed in ED. The patient lost pulses after primary assessment and CPR was initiated with ROSC. Cardiac arrest recurred and the patient was able to be taken to PICU. CXR showed no acute issues and FAST was negative. The patient had a large depressed skull fracture, orbital fracture, and large facial abrasions. The patient was tested and found to be brain dead the following day and care was withdrawn. Referred for donation but did not donate.

Description of PI Process: The case was reviewed at all levels. The issue of initial undertriage was identified and dissected, education and discussion were used to close. Some communication issues were identified and found to not represent significant issues. Death deemed nonpreventable.

Critique: This program did an admirable job of dissecting this case. It is easy for a trauma center to criticize EMS when those practitioners have little experience in the prehospital setting. When caring for a pediatric patient in dire condition, it is easy for the EMS crew to lose situational awareness and not inform the hospital in a timely manner. It is also not unusual for the information to be sparse. It was not clear whether the endotracheal tube was in the wrong place, but because anesthesia was present and the patient was having difficulty they went ahead and replaced the tube under controlled conditions which was appropriate. The EMS agency received feedback on communication with the emergency department and about the endotracheal tube to review the process of placement.

Mature trauma centers view these types of cases as an opportunity to delve deeply into their processes and look for opportunities for improvement. In mature centers that still have a great deal of problems to solve are not usually able to learn from cases such as this. That is why it is imperative for trauma centers to ramp up their PI program quickly and to look toward more mature centers for guidance.

Geriatric Death with Low Injury Severity and Multiple Comorbidities

Case Narrative: This is a 85-year-old male who suffered a ground-level fall. The patient was not a trauma activation. The patient was admitted with severe hyponatremia, delirium tremens, and multiple rib fractures. The patient was admitted to the medicine service. Several days after admission, the patient became agitated. He was given Haldol and Xanax and subsequently suffered a cardiac arrest and despite resuscitation was pronounced dead.

Description of PI Process: The TMD identified several issues: delay in diagnosis and a delay in consultation. The chest radiograph in ED did not identify multiple rib fractures (which led to the delay in consultation), and the patient had a fall in the hospital prior to arrest and this was not properly evaluated. The case was discussed in trauma MDPI, medicine M&M, and ED case review. While no directly reversible error was found, the documentation reflects the discussion of the delays in trauma consultation and misread of CXR.

Critique: These cases are becoming more common as our population ages. Many trauma centers face the dilemma of whether to admit all these injured patients to the trauma service, or allow them to be admitted to medicine due to their overall poor health. First, it is important that the trauma team be consulted on any patient with injuries who will be admitted to a nonsurgical service except in rare circumstances (such as a trivial injury). In this case, the injuries were not properly identified. There should be a PI trail with radiology and EM regarding the missed injury. There should also be investigation about the timeliness of consultation once the injuries were identified.

Dealing with patient falls in the hospital can be vexing. Our philosophy is that if the trauma team would have been consulted if the patient fell at their home and came to the ED, then we should be consulted in the hospital. Many hospitals do not have systems to properly backboard these patients and provide basic EMS care. The trauma program should work with the hospital to develop a consistent system for dealing with serious inpatient falls.

The cause of cardiac arrest in these cases can be difficult to discern. We often attribute these deaths to aspiration, but many patients will have evidence of aspiration after CPR and cardiac arrest for another reason. Autopsies should be obtained if possible.

A Patient with Multiple Life-Threatening Conditions

Case Narrative: A 29-year-old male was shot multiple times. This was a highest-level activation, and the trauma surgeon was present 4 minutes after arrival. The patient had 8–10 gunshot wounds to the abdomen, arms, and legs. In the ED, the patient was briefly responsive, tachycardic, and hypotensive. They attempted to place a central line in the ED and were unsuccessful. The MTP was initiated and the patient was transported to the operating room. The patient underwent laparotomy, repair of small intestinal laceration, control of hepatic bleeding, abdominal packing, and exploration of left brachial artery and vein. The patient was transferred to the SICU in critical condition but went into arrest on arrival and could not be resuscitated.

Description of PI Process: Several issues were identified. First the patient was rushed to the OR without intubation despite anesthesia at the bedside and the patient exhibiting cyanosis. In addition, blood was being transfused through the arm where a brachial vein dissection was later identified. There were also issues with the blood warming device. The minutes from the case presentation and discussion are outstanding. They had documentation of direct communication with involved providers and printed slides from presentations.

Critique: Cases in which the patient requires multiple simultaneous interventions can test the capabilities of any trauma center. The trauma program should simulate, at least at a tabletop discussion, these types of cases to run through the various processes and determine if any changes should be made to procedures.

Another issue in these cases is the problem with hindsight. The patient was taken to the operating room without an airway and that should be investigated; however, the on-scene decision may have been appropriate and the program needs to resist broad rules for these complex situations (such as that all hypotensive patients going to the OR should be intubated). This is a very strong suggestion in our center, but we still provide leeway for the team leader to react to different sets of circumstances. This is why the PI investigation in cases such as this require direct contemporaneous discussions with the providers who cared for the patient.

Here is another similarly complicated case:

Case Narrative: This is a 19-year-old male involved in an MCC. The EMS run sheet is on the chart. This was a highest-level activation and the trauma surgeon was present prior to arrival. The patient was unstable but responded to fluids. Two high-flow access catheters were placed and the FAST was negative. Before CT, blood was administered and a pelvic binder was placed. In CT the patient became more unstable, the massive transfusion protocol was initiated, and the base deficit was worsening. A large hemoperitoneum was seen and the patient was taken to the OR. In the OR, a midline laparotomy was performed but the patient arrested. A thoracotomy was done and the abdomen packed. The patient had a Grade V liver and Grade IV splenic injury. A splenectomy was performed and the liver packed, but the patient remained grossly unstable with recurrent cardiac arrest and finally succumbed.

Description of PI Process: The case was reviewed and was felt to demonstrate questionable management with opportunity for improvement. It was felt the patient spent too much time in the trauma bay, and that the FAST was falsely negative due to the large hemoperitoneum found in the ED. It was felt that the patient should have gone immediately to the OR. The junior attending who was in charge had documented one-on-one meetings with the trauma director to go over opportunities for improvement and other strategies that could have been used to manage the patient.

Critique: The on-scene trauma surgeon had to make a tough decision on whether to take an unstable patient with a negative FAST to the operating room. In this case, the program did an outstanding job identifying the key issues and was rightly concerned about time spent in ED. Documentation of counseling with attending by the trauma director is vital to closing the loop. There is also the opportunity to create simulated cases with similar tough decisions and hold group discussions to align practice.

Index

© The Author(s), under exclusive license to Springer Nature Switzerland AG 2021   137
J. S. Young, *Trauma Center Performance Improvement*,
https://doi.org/10.1007/978-3-030-71048-4